17.99

Visit our website

to find out about other books from Churchill Livingstone
and our sister companies in Harcourt Health Sciences

Register free at

www.harcourt-international.com

and you

* the la   hic
  produ

* the cl   any
  new b

* news

* inform   nces'
  comp
  and N

You will   ring,
informa   e!

Visit th

Back   For
Location:

Search
Order
Journals
Contacts
Careers
Help/FAQ
Register
Home

Virtual Rep

industry and academia.

Corporation.
• Mosby.

Education
- the world's leading publishers of college and
graduate texts and courseware, giving you endless
ideas and teaching solutions.

Register for e-mail updates on new titles

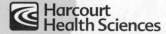

Harcourt
Health Sciences

A Practical Guide to Complaints Handling

For Churchill Livingstone:

Commissioning Editor: Sarena Wolfaard
Project Manager: Jane Shanks
Design Direction: George Ajayi

A Practical Guide to Complaints Handling
In the Context of Clinical Governance

Chris Gunn MA
CG Training, Retford, Nottinghamshire, UK

Foreword by

Michael Buckley
Health Service Commissioner for England, Health Service Ombudsman, London, UK

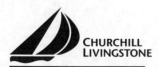
CHURCHILL
LIVINGSTONE

Edinburgh London New York Philadelphia St Louis Sydney Toronto 2001

CHURCHILL LIVINGSTONE

An imprint of Harcourt Publishers Limited

© Harcourt Publishers Limited 2001

 is a registered trademark of Harcourt Publishers Limited

First published 2001

ISBN 0 443 07023 7

British Library Cataloguing in Publication Data
A catalogue record for this book is available from the British Library

Library of Congress Cataloging in Publication Data
A catalog record for this book is available from the Library of Congress

Printed in China

Contents

Foreword

I very much welcome this book, which contains a wealth of helpful advice on the handling and monitoring of NHS complaints.

Complaints are a fact of life. No organisation, and no profession, can avoid them; and it is neither safe nor sensible to ignore or belittle them. Some complaints are trivial: a few complainants are obsessive or malicious. But, for the most part, if complaints are well handled they can have very positive outcomes. Commercial organisations often say that customers who feel that their complaints have been dealt with sympathetically and professionally become their most loyal supporters. Complaints in the NHS often indicate ways in which practice or procedures can be improved, or draw attention to things which may be of no great clinical importance but really matter to patients or their families.

This book covers a great deal of ground and it would be foolish of me to try to summarise it. But I should like to highlight a few key messages.

PERSONAL AND EMOTIONAL ASPECTS

Complaints often stem from very stressful events – serious ill-health or bereavement. Because those making them may be under considerable emotional stress, complaints may contain unreasonable elements or be put in unfair and unreasonable terms. But they must still be assessed objectively.

Complaints can also be very stressful for NHS staff. They may well feel that they have done their best in difficult circumstances, and that their only reward is to be criticised. This reaction, howver understandable, is not helpful. A complaint should not be regarded automatically as an attack on one's personal integrity or professional competence. Something unwelcome has happened – or there would be no complaint – and an explanation needs to be given. Another aspect is that those who are the subject of a complaint can feel isolated and threatened. It is very important that their colleagues should give them sympathy and support.

PRACTICAL ASPECTS

Such things as the layout of a room or the organisation of secretarial support may seem mundane and unimportant. Mundane, perhaps; unimportant, certainly not. A badly organised meeting, for example, can do enormous damage to a complainant's confidence. Many in the NHS who deal with complaints deal with relatively few and have little chance to learn from experience. This book offers a great deal of helpful advice and check-lists.

TECHNICAL AND PROCEDURAL ASPECTS

The NHS complaints procedure is the subject of statutory directions which have the force of law. The requirements of the directions must therefore be observed. But the directions also leave a good deal of discretion. It is at least as important to ensure that discretion is exercised with objectivity, common sense and fairness. In conducting an Independent Review Panel, for example, it is obviously essential to treat the parties to a complaint even-handedly in both substance and manner, to avoid criticising people or organisations which have not had a chance to put their side of a story, and to found conclusions and recommendations firmly on the evidence. Unfortunately, this does not always happen.

Finally, I should like to express my thanks to the author of the book for the fair way in which she has represented the work of my own Office. We do our best to be impartial and objective in considering and investigating complaints; we are much more concerned with the spirit and substance of complaint-handling than with procedural niceties; and we try to minimise the stress that our investigations can impose on complainants and NHS staff alike. But I do understand why some of my former NHS colleagues, when I took up my present post, said to me in the nicest possible way that they hoped never to see me again! I cannot guarantee that result; but I can offer one piece of advice that will greatly increase its probability.

Always give careful thought to communications, but especially during the early stages of a complaint. A dismissive or defensive attitude, or any attempt to get away with less than the whole truth, is all too likely to destroy the complainant's trust. Once destroyed, it is very hard to restore. This greatly increases the likelihood of unsuccessful resolution, discontent with the findings of a Review Panel, and reference to my Office.

London 2000   Michael Buckley

Preface

The correct handling and monitoring of NHS complaints can result in both patient satisfaction and an improvement in the quality of care for future patients. The current system has been in place since April 1996 and the Department of Health has produced guidance documents to supplement the legislation. The aim of this publication is to supplement the existing documentation by giving suggestions and practical examples on all aspects of the complaints process from Local Resolution through to the Select Committee Procedures. From talking to lay chairs, conveners, staff and complainants there is clearly a lack of consistency around the UK and a certain degree of confusion about the different stages of the complaints process. There are subtle differences between the primary care and secondary care legislation and these have been covered in separate sections of the book. Therefore, although there appears to be some duplication between the two sections the changes in approach and the practical examples are different.

Clinical Governance has, rightly, gained more importance in recent years. Where it is recognised that complaints only play a very small (but important) part in the Clinical Governance agenda the issue has been addressed in both the primary and secondary care sections of the book. By linking complaints with Clinical Governance an improvement in the quality of care received by all patients can be achieved.

Many people have assisted with the reading of sections of this book and have offered help and advice; although all are acknowledged in the appendix, a special mention must go to: Rev R. Bennett, Hospital Chaplain, Bassetlaw NHS Trust; A. Corsellis, Professional Interpreter Institute of Linguists; Eric Drake, Investigations Manager, the Health Service Commissioner's Office; Dr Don Gunn; Elaine Read, Consumer Relations Manager, Nottingham Healthcare NHS Trust; and Mr M. Smith, Chief Officer, Bassetlaw Community Health Council.

Retford, Nottinghamshire 2000   Chris Gunn
chris.gunn@cgtraining.demon.co.uk

NHS complaints and clinical governance

SECTION CONTENTS

1

The principles of the complaints procedure

THE COMPLAINANT'S RIGHTS

Anyone making a complaint under the NHS complaints procedure is entitled to three things:

1. A full and complete explanation of what happened and why, given in terminology that the complainant can understand.

2. An apology if there was an error or omission on behalf of the staff.

3. If an error or omission has occurred the complainant should be given information about the action that the organisation has taken, or is proposing to take, to try to prevent it happening again.

Therefore, if errors are identified through the complaints procedure it is essential that there is a process whereby the system can be improved. Although this process may not directly affect the complainant it should reassure them that other patients will not suffer in the same way. It also means that, through the complaints procedure, the quality of patient care should improve for all users of the service.

WHO CAN COMPLAIN?

In order to be investigated under the NHS complaints procedure a complaint must be about NHS services received by an individual patient. The person eligible to make a complaint is the person who was in receipt of the services, that is the patient. It is also possible for someone else to pursue the complaint on behalf of a patient but in order to do this the written consent of the patient must first be obtained. This consent is not required if the complaint is made orally but the moment it is put in writing the consent of the patient must be obtained. If the patient is not able to act then it is possible for someone to pursue a complaint on their behalf without their consent.

If someone has died anyone can make a complaint under the underpinning legislation. However, if the complaints manager does not feel that they are a suitable person then the complaints manager can nominate someone else to act with respect to the complaint.

The NHS complaints procedure deals with NHS complaints and, although other complaints can be investigated by a Health Trust, they do not fall within this system. Examples of these would include: private treatment, theft, abuse, assault and complaints brought by someone who was not directly in receipt of patient care. An example of the last would be if a local councillor complained about the length of time patients were waiting in the out-patient department, or the lack of parking at a practice, or if a neighbour complained about the noise from a residential home.

TIME LIMITS

The object of the complaints procedure is to deal with complaints quickly and accurately and the system has been organised so that this can be done. Built into the process are time limits by which a complainant should have made a complaint. Ideally, complaints should be made as soon as possible after the incident has occurred. It must be within 6 months of the incident or within 6 months from the time that it came to the complainant's notice, providing that not more than 12 months have elapsed since the original incident.

If a complaint is received outside the above time scales it is for the complaints manager to decide whether or not the complaint can be investigated. The two criteria to use to make this decision are that it would have been unreasonable for the complainant to have made the complaint earlier (for example due to a prolonged illness) and that it is still possible to investigate the complaint properly. The organisation may wish to try to answer a complaint on the grounds that it would be in the patient's interest to have the information, but feels that it would be impossible to give a full explanation as some of the information required was not available. It would be advisable in such circumstances to inform the complainant that although the complaint is out of time you are prepared to give an answer, but that this will be done outside the NHS complaints procedure. This course of action is, of course, only acceptable if the complaint is well out of time.

THE STAGES OF THE COMPLAINTS PROCEDURE

The stages in the complaints system are:

• Local Resolution

- The Convening Decision
- The Independent Review Panel
- The Health Service Commissioner (the Ombudsman).

Local Resolution

The vast majority of complaints are resolved at the Local Resolution stage. How Local Resolution is handled is for the individual organisation to decide. Ideally, all staff should be empowered to act on complaints the moment they receive them, as statistics and surveys show that the sooner a complaint is responded to the more likely it is to be resolved. An oral response can be given to an oral complaint and the staff should be aware that this is possible and be able to recognise when they should involve a more senior member of staff to deal with the complaint.

Written complaints have to receive a written response. On the receipt of a written complaint the complaints manager usually initiates an investigation and prepares a written response. The response from the practitioner or the chief executive should then include the result of the investigation, covering all the points raised in the initial complaint, an apology and, if something has gone wrong, an indication of the steps that have been taken to try to prevent it happening again. The initial letter may be followed up with a meeting involving both the complainant and either the complained against or their line manager, depending on the grade of staff involved. Notes should be taken at these meetings and the contents agreed with both parties as to the accuracy of the notes. The meeting is followed by a letter, answering any further questions and supplying extra information as appropriate.

Although not commonly used by Trusts, due to the expertise of the complaints managers, lay conciliation can be used in the Local Resolution process. This is when an external lay person becomes involved in the complaint and acts as an intermediary between the complainant and the complained against. It is useful when the complainant lives a long distance away or during cases of bereavement. Sometimes, if the complainant's perception is that the Trust or practitioner 'killed' their relative or friend and they are therefore not prepared to speak to anyone who works for the organisation, a conciliator is seen as an acceptable, independent person to handle the complaint.

The final letter at the end of Local Resolution must advise the complainant of their rights. A complainant has a right to request (but not to have) an Independent Review Panel and this must be done within 28 days of the final letter following Local Resolution. In order that the request may be considered, the complainant has to say which issues have not been answered during Local Resolution and why they remain dissatisfied.

Clinical Governance

Clinical Governance

The Convening Decision

Any request for an Independent Review Panel is passed to the convener. It is becoming increasingly common for Trusts and Health Authorities to appoint more than one person to act as their convener but at least one of these people must be a non-executive director of the organisation. The convener acknowledges the receipt of the request, takes clinical advice if the complaint is about clinical issues and has to consult with an independent lay chair, who is appointed by the Regional Office of the Department of Health.

The role of the convener and the lay chair is to assess the correspondence and evaluate whether or not the complainant has received a full explanation, which covers all the outstanding issues that they have identified. They also have to assess if an apology is required and, if so, whether it has been given. Finally, if something has gone wrong, they must decide whether it is clear from the correspondence what steps have been taken to try to prevent it happening again.

Depending on the decision they come to, the convener has three options:

- To refer the request back to Local Resolution
- To agree to the request for an Independent Review Panel
- To refuse the request.

Therefore if the convener and lay chair do not understand the explanations given to the complainant they have to decide whether to refer the request back to Local Resolution or to grant the request for a panel. If, on the other hand, they understand the explanations, feel an apology has been given and that there is no further action that can be taken then they can refuse the request for a panel.

If the request is referred back to Local Resolution the convener can suggest what further action could be taken to help to resolve the complaint. The complainant is advised that they can re-request an Independent Review Panel if further Local Resolution does not answer their concerns. If an Independent Review Panel is refused the convener should explain where the outstanding issues have been addressed and advise the complainant that if they remain dissatisfied they have a right to contact the Health Service Commissioner (the Ombudsman).

If it is agreed that an Independent Review Panel should be held then it is the convener's responsibility to write the terms of reference for the panel, which will be based on the issues that remain outstanding from Local Resolution.

The Independent Review Panel

The independent lay chair, the convener and a third lay person form the Independent Review Panel. If there is a clinical content to the complaint then at least two clinical assessors will be appointed to advise the panel on the clinical aspects of the complaint. The guidance produced by the Department of Health leaves the running of the panel to the discretion of the lay chair. This flexibility has the advantage of allowing the panel to take into account the needs of individuals. What is important is that the panel is seen to be fair and to treat both parties equally. The panel is there to investigate events and is not a disciplinary panel. The object is to establish the facts of the case and to make recommendations, if appropriate, to improve the effectiveness or efficiency of the service.

The most common format for the panel is that the clinical assessors review the correspondence and the medical records and prepare a draft report for the panel. The panel and the clinical assessors then meet and interview the complainant first and then the complained against, followed by any witnesses. Immediately after the panel hearing the panel members and the assessors agree the findings of fact, comment on each of the terms of reference and then agree the recommendations. The Health Authority or Trust types up the report and the lay chair and the panel members then agree the final report, which is then sent to the parties concerned.

If, after receiving the report, the complainant remains dissatisfied, or the complained against feels that they were unfairly treated, then they have the right to take the matter up with the Ombudsman.

Following the receipt of the Independent Review Panel report the chief executive of the Trust writes to the complainant and advises them of the action that will be taken to address the recommendations outlined in the panel report. In family health services complaints the chief executive writes to the practitioner requesting that they respond to the complaint and outline the actions taken.

The Health Service Commissioner (the Ombudsman)

The complainant has a right to go to the Health Service Commissioner (the Ombudsman) if the convener refuses their request for an Independent Review Panel or if they remain dissatisfied at the end of the Independent Review Panel. The Ombudsman reviews the request and decides whether or not to investigate. If it appears that an investigation may be warranted then they may request that the organisation supplies information about how the complaint was handled and any further information that may help to make a final decision. The Ombudsman is interested to see that the correct procedure has been followed. For example, at the Convening Decision stage, did the convener consult with a lay chair and did they take appropriate clinical advice if it was a clinical complaint?

If the Ombudsman decides to investigate, all the parties involved in the complaints process are interviewed and a report is written and published.

Clinical Governance

THE INTERFACE WITH DISCIPLINARY ACTION, LEGAL ACTION AND CLINICAL GOVERNANCE

It is very clear that the disciplinary process must be kept separate from the complaints process. In addition, it is not the role of either the complaints manager or the convener to decide if disciplinary action needs to be taken. In Trust complaints, if either the complaints manager or the convener feels that there is an indication that there is a prima facie case for disciplinary action they should refer the matter to the member(s) of the Trust management team responsible for such actions. If it is decided that disciplinary action is to be taken then the complaints procedure must stop with regard to that aspect of the complaint and the complainant informed that disciplinary action has been taken. In primary care complaints the complaint could be referred to the professional regulatory body, the NHS tribunal or the police. Only following the receipt of an Independent Review Panel Report can the Health Authority's reference panel decide whether or not disciplinary proceedings should be initiated.

If a complainant instructs a solicitor to take legal action then the complaints procedure must stop. It is important to clarify that the complainant has instructed a solicitor, as a letter from a solicitor may or may not mean that legal action has been started. Currently, it is unlikely that a complainant will receive legal aid unless they have been through the NHS complaints procedure. Complainants are therefore usually advised by solicitors to follow the complaints procedure and then return to them if they still wish to pursue legal action.

Clinical Governance will become more important as the systems are developed. Many organisations set up panels to review the complaints procedure, to look not only at how complaints are handled but also at areas of concern and trends in complaints. If an organisation is to benefit from its complaints procedure it will need a method of learning from complaints and will need to take positive action if problems are identified through the process.

2

Understanding complainants

It must be emphasised that all complaints must be fully investigated. The information in this chapter must not be used as an excuse for not handling a complaint correctly. It has been written in an attempt to help staff understand what is different about handling NHS complaints. It is very difficult and stressful to handle someone who is angry and appears not to understand what you are saying. Hopefully, after reading this chapter, staff will have gained an insight into why people may be behaving as they are.

Anger, and the need to complain, can arise from the complainant revisiting an earlier bereavement or other emotional episode that was ignored or denied when it originally occurred. In this case the complaint and associated anger may be nothing to do with the incident being complained about, and staff should bear this possibility in mind. Staff need to understand that although the anger may be directed at them they may not be to blame and it may not be as a result of anything that they have done. In other words, anger is sometimes not directed at them personally but at the position they represent, and the complainant will require patience and understanding to help them get through what, for them, is a very traumatic experience.

WHAT MAKES NHS COMPLAINTS DIFFERENT?

Unfortunately, one of the things that it is not possible to do under the NHS complaints procedure is to turn the clock back. Although it may be possible to take a patient back to surgery and possibly put right an error, if a patient has died it is not possible to bring them back to life again. When a member of staff has been rude or dismissive to a patient an apology can be given, but it is not possible to unsay words once they have been said.

Unfortunately, some complainants wish to see members of staff disciplined and, in some extreme cases, 'struck off'. They feel that if they had been negligent at work they could lose their job and therefore that the same standards should apply in the Health Service. This is an understandable reaction and, if the complaint is serious enough to warrant either disciplinary action or referral to the appropriate professional body, the NHS tribunal or the police, then this should be initiated by the Trust or Health Authority and the complainant should be advised that the action has been taken. The problems arise when the member of staff acted appropriately, given the information that was available at the time the patient was being treated. If a patient does not have the signs and symptoms associated with the diagnosis of a particular disease and the tests undertaken show no abnormality, then it is impossible for a disease to be detected. In such a scenario, in the patient's view the doctor failed to diagnose an illness but the doctor's view is that they tried hard but were unable to make a diagnosis, and therefore were not to blame. The only way to resolve this type of conflict is to explain fully what tests were given and why, and also what symptoms the doctor would have expected to see, and to indicate that they were not present.

In some more serious complaints the emotional state of the complainant has to be taken into account. When a complaint involves, for example, the sudden death of a young person both the staff and relatives feel the loss. Both parties tend to think 'if only'. For example, if only …:

- …I had sent for the doctor earlier
- …I had visited the patient during the afternoon
- …I had started the drugs earlier
- …I had told the doctor about…
- …I had realised how ill they were
- …I had not gone to that meeting
- …I had told them I loved them
- …We had not quarrelled last week
- …I had not decided to operate on the other patient first
- …I had not let them play outside.

There are many more examples of what both staff and relatives think but often do not say. In other areas where complaints are dealt with it is relatively easy to 'put right the wrong'. For example, if a piece of equipment breaks down the equipment can either be mended or replaced. This option is not available if someone has lost a loved one or if a patient has suffered irreparable brain damage or spinal damage resulting in paralysis.

WHY DO PEOPLE COMPLAIN?

Surveys indicate that most complainants want the NHS to recognise and acknowledge when errors have happened. They want an explanation for what has happened and, if something has gone wrong, they want a proper apology. They also want to know that what happened to them or their loved one will not happen to someone else. Therefore complainants wish to know what steps have been taken to prevent the problem recurring and from that they want the NHS to learn from complaints. Some complainants want staff to be disciplined if an error has occurred and a small number are looking for financial compensation.

Some complaints involve the sudden death of a patient. It should be remembered that feelings associated with normal grieving can result in a feeling of anger and in some instances this anger can be displaced or directed towards another person. In other instances it can be directed towards staff, which can result in a complaint. It must be emphasised that if a person has died something may have gone wrong and the complaint must be investigated thoroughly. But staff need to understand that complainants may be very angry and have difficulty in absorbing what people say as a result of the grieving process they are going through.

THE EFFECT OF BEREAVEMENT

Bereavement is defined as the normal human reaction to loss and, as a result, medical situations other than death can result in a feeling of loss and bereavement:

- Loss of a body part (e.g. a limb or a breast)
- Loss of body image (e.g. due to trauma or disease)
- Loss of senses (e.g. hearing, eyesight)
- Loss of function (e.g. paralysis or breathing problems)
- Relative admitted to care (e.g. due to dementia, terminal cancer).

People react differently to loss; some of the more common reactions that are associated with complaints handling include:

- Anger
- Guilt
- Shock, numbness and disbelief.

Other reactions can include:

- Denial (or an unwillingness to accept that a loved one has died)
- Bargaining (when a person knows a loved one has died but feels that they can either say something or do something to change what has taken place)
- Acceptance (this can happen when the person feels relieved that a person is no longer suffering)
- Depression (due to being left alone or a feeling of being unable to cope).

Clinical Governance

Clinical Governance

Anger

Anger is a natural reaction to loss. In some instances it is turned against the person who has died, in other instances it is directed towards people who the bereaved blames for the death. These people can include carers, doctors and nurses. Occasionally, this anger is directed at a member of staff who has been particularly kind and supportive to the family, probably because they also feel let down by a person whom they had trusted.

Guilt

Guilt is another natural reaction. Anecdotal evidence indicates that a proportion of the more complex complaints are instigated by a relative who lives a distance away. Such complaints are often associated with a group of relatives who live near and who visited the patient on a regular basis. The close relatives may often say how pleased they were with the treatment offered but the distant relative remains unhappy. People who live at a distance and lead busy lives cannot easily assess the severity of their relative's illness. They may want to visit but circumstances may not permit this. They may contact the patient or the ward regularly but do not get the impression that it is necessary to visit as the situation does not appear, to them, to be life threatening. They may (or may not) be in contact with the relatives who live locally and, again, may not have a full picture given of the situation. Consequently, when the patient dies they are left with the feeling of 'if only'.

Shock, numbness and disbelief

Although in themselves the feelings of shock, anger and disbelief may not result in a person making a complaint, they can affect the way that people react when information is given to them. They may have difficulty in absorbing what people say and, later, will sometimes say that they were not given information. For this reason, any discussions or meetings with a relative who has recently suffered a loss should be followed up with a letter that summarises the questions asked and the answers and explanations given. The person will be able to re-read the letter at their leisure and there is therefore a greater chance that they will be able to absorb more of the information given.

Difficulties occur when people become 'stuck' in one of the normal reactions to loss. They can become locked into a particular stage and are unable to move on. In these instances a particular reaction may become extremely intense and may actually prevent a person from functioning normally. This can result in almost obsessive behaviour, which can very occasionally be seen in patients who are pursuing a complaint. Complainants sometimes become locked onto something that has happened in the hospital, or during treatment, and refuse to accept rational explanations or to acknowledge that staff have admitted that an error has occurred. On talking to the complainant it is often very difficult to find out what they really want to happen as a result of their complaint or what action would satisfy them. These complainants may require professional help to assist them in coming to terms with their grief but unfortunately any offer of assistance often results in a refusal and an accusation that staff are not taking their complaint seriously.

Clinical Governance

3

Supporting complainants

THE ROLE OF THE COMMUNITY HEALTH COUNCIL

The Community Health Councils (CHCs) often describe themselves as the patient's friend. Each CHC is made up of representatives from voluntary organisations, local councillors and people appointed by the appropriate Regional Office of the NHS Executive. The CHC members oversee the work of the permanent staff and perform monitoring and inspection visits to local Trusts. Providing information about the National Health Service to the general public is a large part of their role and, although complaints handling is not one of the statutory functions of the CHCs, it has been recognised as a key role of CHCs in official guidance.

There are about 200 CHCs in England and Wales and the Association of Community Health Councils for England and Wales (ACHCEW) publishes a directory and can provide contact details for organisations in specific localities. Information can be obtained from:

ACHCEW, Earlsmead House, 30 Drayton Park, London N5 1PB
Tel. 020 7609 8405

The CHCs pride themselves on their independence from the main-stream Health Service and are ideally situated to offer independent and confidential advice to people wishing to make a complaint. It is usually the staff of the CHC who undertake the complaints work, rather than the voluntary members.

The level of service, help and advice to complainants will vary from council to council as many have only two or three members of staff and very large workloads. CHCs will be able to offer complainants some or all of the following, on a confidential basis:

- Leaflets about the complaints procedure
- Verbal information and advice about making a complaint
- Assistance with the drafting of letters of complaint
- Someone to accompany the complainant to Local Resolution meetings
- Assistance with drafting letters requesting an Independent Review Panel
- Someone to make telephone calls on the complainant's behalf
- Someone to accompany the complainant to Independent Review Panels
- Information about other organisations that could give help and advice, for example bereavement care
- Assistance with contacting the Health Service Commissioner and with any subsequent support if an investigation takes place
- Assistance with referrals to any other official bodies, for example the General Medical Council or the police.

As they are seen as independent organisations, complainants will often contact their CHC for help and advice. Although some complainants are reluctant to make contact, those that do, report high levels of satisfaction in the service they are offered. Unfortunately, not all Health Authorities. Trusts and primary care practitioners mention the CHC to complainants in their literature and correspondence.

In addition to assisting complainants, CHC officers may undertake consumer satisfaction surveys and assist with the monitoring of complaints. Meetings between Trust, Health Authority or primary care staff and CHC officers can be invaluable and lead to improvements in the service offered to complainants and, therefore, through them, to patients. The CHC staff can often feed back comments from complainants and indicate areas where improvements can be made. As meetings are a two-way process, they can also be a mechanism for improving the quality of information that is presented by the complainants. A simple example would be to encourage complainants to list and number their complaints and, ideally, present them in date order. This would enable a clear response to be sent and to ensure that all areas of concern are covered in the response.

THE USE OF PATIENT ADVOCATES

Some of the larger Trusts employ a member of staff with the title 'patient's advocate'. The role of this member of staff is to deal with complaints as early as possible, ideally before the complainant leaves the hospital. If a complaint is made the advocate is paged and, if possible, goes to the ward or the department to speak to the complainant. The advocate tries to deal with the complaint at once but, if further investigation is required, takes details, investigates on behalf of the complainant and provides information for the response letter sent by the chief executive.

It could be argued that the above description is that of the complaints manager, and in some Trusts that may be true. What is important is the speed of the response. Research has shown that many complaints can be dealt with effectively if they are responded to quickly. It could be argued that the term 'patient's advocate' gives a much more positive message to complainants than 'complaints manager' or 'customer care manager'. Also, patients tend to regard the 'patient's advocate' as at least trying to solve their problems, rather than as a defendant of the organisation complained against. What is vital for the role to be successful is that the advocate can respond quickly to complaints, therefore any additional work that they are given should enable them to give priority to complaints handling.

THE USE OF INTERPRETERS

When handling complaints it is essential that the person dealing with the complaint fully understands what the other person is complaining about. Wherever possible, interpreters should be used to make sure that the facts are accurately and precisely recorded. In order to do this anyone acting as an interpreter should have a high degree of competence in the language and be able to understand the context in which they are working. A list of qualified interpreters can be obtained from:

The Institute of Linguists, Saxon House, 48 Southwark Road, London SE1 1UN
Tel. 020 7940 3100
Web site www.iol.org.uk

It is worth considering using professional interpreters at the Local Resolution stage to make sure that the person making the complaint is listened to and that they receive a clear explanation of what has happened and full answers to all their questions.

There are strong arguments in favour of using professional interpreters, as they:

- Have a high level of knowledge and understanding of both the culture and the language they are interpreting for
- Have the skills and techniques to accurately transfer information from one language to another
- Observe an enforceable code of conduct that includes the need for confidentiality and impartiality.

As there are requirements to provide an equal service irrespective of language, culture, etc. the use of a professional interpreter may well reduce the chance of litigation. Therefore the use of professionals may well prove to be cheaper in the long run.

If using relatives or bilingual members of staff to act as interpreters, staff need to be aware that the questions should come from the complainant and should check that the replies are being translated for them. It is very easy for the interpreter to slip into the role of advocate and ask the questions they want to have answered, rather than those of the complainant. In addition, they may not have all the skills or understanding of a professional interpreter.

ASSISTING COMPLAINANTS WITH A DISABILITY

The Council on Tribunals has produced a checklist and code of practice on 'Access for Disabled People Using the Tribunal System'. Although, as its name suggests, the principles contained in the publication are concerned with access to tribunals, they also apply to any public building or meeting.

The document is written on the principle that all citizens have the right of access whether they are disabled or non-disabled. It provides a list of contact addresses, a glossary of disability terms and a guide to disability etiquette, which has been produced by the Royal Association for Disability and Rehabilitation (RADAR).

The list below highlights issues to consider and makes some practical points.

Car parking

- Is disabled car parking available?
- Is it signposted?
- Is there space for wheelchair users to leave and enter their vehicles?
- Do your letters and publications indicate the availability and location of the disabled car parking?
- Is the parking close to the entrance the drivers will use?
- If the above does not apply, how and where can the users park?

Public transport

- Is public transport available?
- Do your letters and publications indicate its availability?
- How far is it to the entrance people will use?
- Do you provide information about local Dial-a-Ride or firms providing accessible taxis?
- Are there access problems and, if so, have people been told about them? For example at the local station.
- Do you provide a large-scale map showing the entrance and location of the premises used?

Signposting

- Is the venue clearly signposted?
- Are the signs large, of sufficient contrast and written in lower case for the visually impaired?
- Is Braille signposting required?

The entrance

- Are there steps? Is the edge clearly marked and do they have a non-slip surface?
- Is there a ramp of the correct gradient? (No steeper than 1 in 15 if the flights are no longer than 10 m or 1 in 12 if they are no longer than 5 m.)
- Are there handrails of the correct height and with a surface that aids gripping them?
- Is the accessible entrance in the same place as the entrance for non-disabled people?
- Is there an entry phone? Can it be used by someone in a wheelchair?
- If there is a revolving door, is there an adjacent door?
- Can someone in a wheelchair or on crutches open the doors?
- Are the doors wide enough to allow wheelchair access (a minimum clear opening of 750 mm)?

Toilets

- Are there toilets near the room being used for the meeting?
- Do they comply with the relevant British Standard?
- Are they properly maintained?

Additional facilities

- Can you accommodate a signer, helper, etc?
- Are there facilities for guide dogs?
- Are refreshments available? Do you provide for people with special diets?
- Is first-aid available or obtainable?
- Is there an accessible public telephone? Can it be operated from a wheelchair? Is there an induction loop and/or a volume control?

At the meeting

- Is the room far from the lift or waiting area?
- Are the acoustics adequate?

- Is an induction loop fitted?
- If requested, could you provide an interpreter for any language? For the deaf?
- Could hand-written documents be retyped?
- If required, could papers or letters be available in large print, tape or Braille?
- Does any furniture in the room restrict access?
- Are there a range of seats available so people with different disabilities can be comfortably seated?

General behaviour

- How do the staff behave towards people with disabilities?
- Has disability awareness training been given?

COMPLAINANTS WITH LEARNING DIFFICULTIES

Complainants with learning difficulties have the same rights as others in society. Given time, patience and the right environment they are often able to express their concerns. It is acceptable to appoint patient advocates to work with the complainant and to make sure that all their issues have been addressed and that they understand the responses given. Unfortunately, people who are unable to express themselves clearly sometimes do not get the same standard of care as the more articulate members of society.

Any discussion should take place with the minimum number of people present so as not to either frighten or intimidate the person making the complaint. It should be remembered that often their thinking process is much slower and therefore care should be taken not to put 'words into their mouth'; people should be prepared to wait a little longer than normal for a verbal response.

When distressed, people are sometimes unable to articulate their fears and therefore resort to shouting, which may be seen as being aggressive rather than an expression of frustration. Often, by speaking quietly to the complainant, encouraging them to sit down and showing that you are prepared to listen to them, you will help them to calm down and progress can be made.

SUPPORTING THE BEREAVED

Understandably, the loss of a loved one, the diagnosis of a terminal illness or the loss of a body part may result in a complaint being made about the treatment received. As was mentioned in Chapter 2, anger and guilt are two of the common reactions to loss and the anger may well be directed at hospital staff.

All complaints should be dealt with quickly and sympathetically but this is even more important when a person is grieving. In some instances the use of a bereavement councillor during the early stages of a complaint can assist the complainant by providing them with a trained person to talk to. Unfortunately, people often say that they do not wish to have counselling, although they sometimes reconsider after reflection. Providing them with names and addresses of local contacts or offering the opportunity to arrange a meeting with a bereavement care worker may enable them to access the services either immediately or at a later date. If useful addresses are provided at the end of the complaints leaflet the inclusion of details of bereavement care will be an opportunity to provide this information in an unobtrusive way. All Trusts have access to a hospital chaplain and a discussion between the complaints manager, the hospital chaplain and a bereavement care worker will assist the complaints manager to understand the bereavement process and to be able to understand how and when the bereavement care services can be offered.

NHS

Clinical Governance

4

Monitoring and Clinical Governance

COMPLAINT REVIEWS

What should be recorded?

The recording of statistics alone is insufficient for the accurate monitoring of complaints; it is also necessary to record the content of the complaints so that trends and clinical areas or individuals that are receiving a higher than average number of complaints can be identified. Wherever possible, oral complaints should also be recorded as they may indicate 'minor grumbles' that, individually, do not appear to be important but collectively can show areas where improvements can be made both cheaply and effectively.

There is a tendency just to examine and review complaints. This can give a distorted view of the work of the organisation and thought should therefore be given to recording both complaints and compliments. By doing this, a more realistic judgement can be made about the work of a particular person or department. A very simple and effective Trust form, entitled Complaints, Comments and Compliments, can provide three sections in which people can record comments under the appropriate heading. This simple method allows the person completing the form to decide which category their comment comes under and then enables a database to be collated for all three areas.

One of the problems encountered by relying on numbers alone to assess the effectiveness and efficiency of a service is that organisations that openly advertise their complaints system and make forms freely available for people to make comments will attract a far greater number of complaints than those that are not quite as open and forthcoming.

Who should monitor complaints?

Under the legislation, Trusts are responsible for monitoring complaints and preparing quarterly reports about the nature and volume of complaints. In addition, an annual report has to be published and sent to the Regional Office, the Local Health Authority and the local CHC(s). In primary care, the number of complaints received by individual practices should be sent to Health Authorities on a quarterly basis for monitoring purposes. The Health Authority has to produce an annual report on complaints handling, a copy of which has to be sent to the NHS Executive and all relevant CHCs.

Whether a specific complaints monitoring group is organised or whether complaints are reviewed under the quality, risk management or clinical governance arrangements is up to the individual organisation. The involvement of non-executive directors in the evaluation can bring an independent perspective to the process and some Trusts and Health Authorities involve members of the CHC and also survey complainants to get their views.

What should be monitored?

It is important that complaints are seen as a way of improving the quality of service provided. Unfortunately, in some places and by some staff they are regarded as a criticism of an individual and therefore staff feel threatened by them. Support and advice should be available to staff and training may be required to ensure that staff feel confident about handling complaints and do not take them personally. An open and honest environment will make the recording, and therefore the monitoring and improvement in services, more effective.

A systematic approach is needed for complaints monitoring. The information collected should include:

- The category the complaint falls into
- Which unit, department or ward is involved
- If an individual member of staff was involved
- How the complaint was handled
- The outcome of the complaint
- Whether action is required following the complaint
- Whether or not the action has taken place
- Whether the lessons learnt can be applied to other areas of the Trust or practice.

The category the complaint falls into

The headings used will vary between individual units but most will certainly include: oral and written communication, record keeping, the type and quality of patient information, the manner and attitude of staff, waiting and appointment times, and telephone access. They could also include such areas as car parking, signposting, catering, cleanliness/hygiene, quality of written information, etc.

Which unit, department, ward or member of staff is involved?

Recording which departments or individuals are receiving complaints can help to identify trends, including unacceptable changes in practice or routine. If certain department or individuals are attracting a higher than average number of complaints then further investigation will be required to identify the reason for this.

How was the complaint handled?

This could include the time taken for a complaint to be resolved but a more useful guide is for the use of random sampling to look at the quality of the responses that are being sent out. Some organisations give a list of complaints received, identified only by a number. A nominated person, for example, the senior partner, the clinical governance lead, the medical director, the nursing director or a non-executive director, selects a number at random and then reviews the complaint documentation. The person or persons would look at the response with regard to layout, clarity of information, accuracy of information, the fullness of the response and whether or not the aims of the Local Resolution process have been met.

The outcome of the complaint

Just because a complainant has not continued with a complaint does not mean that they were satisfied with the outcome. Responses to complaints can be examined by addressing the following questions:

- Would the person evaluating the complaint have been satisfied with the answer?
- Could the responses have been improved?
- Were there lessons that could be learnt?
- Was any action required on behalf of the organisation or individual?
- Was the action taken?

THE DISSEMINATION OF INFORMATION

Complaints can be used to indicate improvements to services across the whole organisation but how often is this done? How effectively is the information communicated and are all staff aware of any changes and how and when they should be implemented? Individual letters or e-mails, management meetings, newsletters or bulletins can be used to communicate information. If procedures have changed, complainants often appreciate being told of the changes that have taken place as a result of their complaint. It is appreciated that, due to monetary constraints, it is not always possible to implement major changes but many complaints are to do with poor communication and the lack of recorded information. Consideration needs to be given to the most effective way of encouraging staff to change unacceptable practices. Staff are more likely to improve their communication skills and record keeping if they understand the likely consequences of their actions and, by publishing anonymous examples of complaints, concrete examples can be given.

ACTION FOLLOWING AN INDEPENDENT REVIEW PANEL

If a complaint results in an Independent Review Panel then it is usual for recommendations to be made by the panel.

Action by the chief executive

The chief executive writes to the complainant stating whether or not the Trust accepts the recommendations made by the panel and what action it proposed as a result of the recommendations. In primary care, the chief executive writes to the practitioner with a copy of the final report and invites the practitioner to respond to any recommendations directly to the complainant. Although it is not mandatory to copy this letter to the panel members, by doing so, they will receive an indication that the time and effort that they have put in to the panel has resulted in some action. From the panel members' perspective it does help to 'round off' their work in a much more satisfactory way than if they are not kept informed.

Follow-up and review

Although the chief executive or the practitioner writes to complainants following an Independent Review Panel, is there an in-house mechanism for informing complainants when the agreed action will be taken? Equally, is the complainant told when the changes have been implemented? By not informing others of action taken as a result of complaints, the organisation is vulnerable to the accusation that it is not taking action, and therefore complaints, seriously. If there is an open and transparent mechanism in place for keeping complainants informed the complainants are more likely to feel that they have achieved something.

Involving complainants

One way of monitoring complaints is through surveys, which can be done by the practitioner, the Trust, or in conjunction with the CHC. This can help to give an indication of whether or not complainants have been satisfied with the responses they have received or if they just became overwhelmed by the process. If an organisation suddenly receives a large number of comments about a particular area of service these can be addressed by inviting all complainants to a meeting to discuss their concerns. This 'focus group' approach allows concerns to be aired and can identify very effectively the problem areas. It also publicly demonstrates that the organisation is prepared to take complaints seriously and to act on peoples' concerns.

Clinical Governance

5

Specialist complaints handling

Complaints should always be investigated thoroughly and especially so in those areas that fall into the category of 'specialist complaints'. These include complaints connected with bereavement, serial or vexatious complaints and mental health complaints. These complaints should always be investigated carefully as it is very easy for health professionals to fall into the trap of thinking that it is the complainant's fault that something has gone wrong, and not the fault of the staff.

Because of the emotional state that some complainants are in they sometimes have difficulty expressing themselves and fully outlining their concerns. In some instances they do not know what they are complaining about, all they know is that they are unhappy with what has happened to them. Sometimes the staff are unable to give these people the time they deserve and fail to understand that what the staff describe as aggression may well be a cover for fear and frustration at the inability to express those fears in any other way.

Staff need to consider that a complainant's behaviour may be the result of an underlying medical condition, for example mental illness or dementia, the effect of drugs or alcohol or a personality disorder. In addition, there could be physical factors such as pain, hunger or sleep deprivation, which could be due to their illness or home circumstances.

If the complainant is or has been a patient at the hospital, the involvement of the clinician dealing with them may prove beneficial. In all instances, wherever possible, the well-being of the patient should come first. A change of drug dosage, a review of medication or the referral to other agencies, including bereavement care, counselling or social services may assist the patient and be more effective than allowing them to get into a cycle of complaints correspondence that appears to have no end point.

Bereavement has been addressed in Chapters 2 and 3 and this chapter will therefore concentrate on serial complainants and mental health complaints.

SERIAL COMPLAINANTS

Serial complainants can cause enormous problems for organisations both in the form of staff time and the emotional stress for staff that can result from dealing with the complainant. Fortunately, most organisations do not have large numbers of complainants that fall into this category but the frequency is such that most people working in the field of complaints will come across at least one such person during their career. Unfortunately, some of the larger Trusts may have more than their fair share of this type of complainant.

Frequent complainers

These people tend to make frequent complaints but each complaint is distinct and separate from the previous one. They may be known to other organisations, which are also on the receiving end of complaints from the same person. With this type of complainant each complaint must be investigated and a response given. However, it may not always be necessary to conduct a very detailed and extensive investigation. The amount of time taken to investigate the complaint should be determined by the type of complaint and not by the type of complainant. Therefore in some instances only a brief response may be required whilst in others a more detailed response becomes necessary.

Serial complainants policy

It is recommended that Trusts and Health Authorities have an agreed policy on dealing with these complainants. This should include a definition as to the type of person that would fall into the category and a procedure for dealing with the complaints. Included in the policy should be a recognition of the effect such patients have on staff and clear mechanisms should be in place to provide staff support. It is also recommended that any policy should be instigated only in exceptional circumstances and then only with the approval of both the chief executive and the chair of the Health Authority or Trust. In this way there is a safeguard to ensure that the policy is used only as a last resort.

Definition of a serial complainant

A serial complainant is someone who:

- Is in frequent contact with the complaints department. They make contact every day and in some instances more frequently either by telephone or by physically calling in to the department.
- Will attend or telephone even though they have been given a date for a meeting or have been told that the Trust or Health Authority will write to them by a specific date.
- Has been aggressive or abusive to staff. This could include the complaints staff, parties involved with the treatment and care of the patient and other staff including receptionists, telephonists and senior managers.
- Is adamant that they have not had a response when a number of meetings have taken place to answer their specific questions and a large amount of correspondence has been sent in an attempt to address their concerns.
- Challenges written documentation by claiming that the records have been altered. Refuses to accept contemporaneous notes even though different people have made them.
- When a response is received from the organisation, immediately responds by either raising new concerns or presenting an old problem in a different way. In this way the complaint is kept moving but it is difficult to complete due to the increasing number of new issues being raised.
- Changes the complaints or what they want to achieve part way through the complaint.
- Tries to manipulate the complaint by:
  — complaining about the member of staff dealing with the complaint
  — dictating who they will and will not speak to, for example wanting to speak directly to the chair of the Trust or the chief executive of the Health Authority
  — stating that they wish to meet with a person and then either refusing to arrange a date for a meeting or not turning up after a meeting has been arranged
  — making the same, or a slightly different complaint to other people, for example, the Press, the local Member of Parliament, the Health Secretary, the Prime Minister, the Queen, either concurrently or consecutively.
- Seeks an unrealistic outcome and intends to continue until that outcome is achieved. Examples could include wanting to have a member of staff sacked or operations carried out on demand.
- Complains about an event that has happened in the past, which cannot be changed.

It should be noted that the complainant may or may not fulfil all the above criteria but the policy should indicate the number of the criteria that have to be met before the complainant can be categorised as being a serial complainant. If, for example, the complainant had also written to their

Member of Parliament they would not be classified as a serial complainant because they may have been unaware of the complaints procedure and how to access it.

Dealing with abuse

Staff should not be expected to have to put up with abuse either on the telephone or in person. Clear procedures should therefore be in place so that staff are aware of the action that should be taken when faced with an abusive situation. If someone is being abusive on the telephone the staff member can say that they are not prepared to listen to abuse and will put the telephone down if the abuse continues. If the caller persists in abusing the staff then they should state that they are ending the call and put the telephone down. A record should immediately be made of what was said and the timing of the call. The incident should then be reported to the line manager.

If the calls are repeated, the telephonists or secretaries should be instructed to terminate the call once the caller has identified themselves, again a record should be made of all incidents and a report made to the line manager. The complainant should be advised, in writing, that staff have been instructed not to take calls and that all future communication will be in writing only.

If the complainant is aggressive during an interview they again should be warned that the behaviour is not acceptable and a short break should be taken. If the aggression continues then the interview should be terminated and the complainant asked to leave. As before, the event should be reported and documented.

Threatened assault

If it is thought that staff are at risk from violence then it is important that steps are taken to safeguard the staff. When interviewing a potentially violent person, ensure that the staff member will not become trapped in the room and that they can get help if a problem arises. A calm atmosphere helps and anything that could be used as a weapon should be removed from the room. Wherever possible, encourage the person to sit down and remember it is much more difficult for a person to get out of a low, soft chair than a high solid one! The complainant should be advised that if there is any suggestion of risk or if they become threatening the interview will be terminated. Hospital security staff may be contacted and consideration should be given to arranging for them to be available and in position so that they can be called on to assist if necessary. If it is thought that staff would be at risk then the interview should not take place. Again, any incident must be documented and reported.

Any threats to staff must be taken seriously and if it is thought that staff may be at risk both in the hospital and at home then steps should be taken to ensure they are protected.

Suggested procedures for handling serial complainants

The chief executive and the chair of the Health Authority or Trust should agree that the complaint falls into the category of a serial complaint. The decision should be recorded and the reason for the decision should also be noted.

It is important to check that the complainant's concerns have been fully investigated and that the information has been sent to the complainant. The complainant should be encouraged to request an Independent Review Panel so that the documentation can be checked by the convener, an independent lay chair and a clinical adviser. This would then mean that the initial complaints handling had been scrutinised by independent people and if, in their opinion, the aims of local resolution had been met, the request would be refused. The complainant would be advised of their right to contact the Ombudsman in the normal way. If the complainant had not had a full explanation then the complaint would either be referred back to Local Resolution or on to a panel in the normal way.

If the complainant is not prepared to request a panel or insists on raising the same issue again, they should be advised that as the chief executive has responded fully to the points raised, the matter is now closed. They could also be told that no further correspondence would be entered into unless they have a new complaint, which is separate from the original complaint. They could also be advised that staff will no longer deal with the complainant over the telephone and that they have a right to contact the Ombudsman if they remain dissatisfied.

If the complainant replies again, the next response could inform the complainant that the letter they sent had been received and the contents noted. A copy of the letter answering the complaint could be enclosed with a statement to the effect that there is nothing further to add to that letter.

In very extreme cases, where abusive behaviour continues, complainants may have to be informed that the Trust or Health Authority's solicitors may have to become involved. As a last resort, a writ for defamation could be issued or an injunction made, but legal advice should be sought and the Regional NHS Executive informed before this action is taken.

If a policy is in place then there will be an open procedure for dealing with this problem area. It is far better to have the policy in place before a serial complaint is received than to try and write one in the middle of dealing with the problem.

Staff support

Unfortunately, those not handling complaints do not realise that dealing with complaints on a regular basis can be very exhausting and stressful for the staff involved. Senior managers should be on the look-out for signs of stress in their staff and an opportunity should be given at regular intervals for staff to discuss problem areas with their line manager. Staff who have been dealing with a serial complainant or a particularly complex and time-consuming complaint may need external support. Some Trusts and Health Authorities have provided access to a counselling service for staff, to be used as and when required, and others have encouraged staff to use the occupational health scheme. Good complaints managers can and do save organisations a considerable amount of money and medical staff time by effectively dealing with complaints so any money spent on their health and well-being can be viewed as being a very good investment.

MENTAL HEALTH COMPLAINTS

Patients with mental health problems pose particular challenges to staff dealing with their complaints. It is helpful if someone with a clinical background is responsible for seeing all complaints from patients with mental health problems as they can bring a clinical perspective to the complaints handling and therefore help to reach an understanding of what the complainant is trying to achieve. It is still imperative that all complaints are treated in the same way and the fact that a complainant has mental health problems should not stop them from having their concerns answered fully. Some patients and relatives fear that there may be reprisals and that their treatment may be compromised if they complain. Consideration could be given to ways in which comments could be received, possibly anonymously. One example would be to use the type of form mentioned on page 23, with three headings – complaints, comments, compliments – and a space for patient details. This, combined with a number of 'post boxes' around the Trust, would enable patients or relatives to make comments anonymously if they wished.

Patients with mental health problems may have difficulty in identifying what their problem actually is and often the complaint that they present initially does not relate to their actual complaint. Time taken immediately after the complaint has been received can often pay dividends. If the patient holds delusional beliefs it can be dangerous for a complaints manager to interview the patient and therefore advice should be taken from the clinical staff in the first instance. If the clinical staff agree that the complainant could be interviewed by the complaints manager it may be possible, through the interview, to determine the events that have led to the complaint and whether a written response or a meeting is the best way of handling the complaint.

Written responses

Written responses should be clearly laid out, perhaps using the questions asked by the complainant as headings in the response. In this way each question will then have an answer underneath and it will be clear that answers have been given. All correspondence should receive a response, even for letters that state:

The treatment I received at the hospital was fine but I am writing to complain about the terrible weather I was faced with when leaving the hospital.

The response should indicate that the Trust was pleased that the complainant was satisfied with the treatment they received and sorry about the weather, but unfortunately this was beyond the control of the Trust. In this way the letter is responded to and there is an acknowledgement that the weather was bad.

Meetings

If, following a written response from the chief executive or practitioner, the patient remains dissatisfied, a meeting could be held.

Care should be taken when structuring meetings to make sure that they are held in a safe and unthreatening environment for all parties. Wherever possible, the number of people present at any one time should be kept to a minimum to enable clear responses to be given. Some Trusts run a patient advocacy scheme where, if the patient has made a request for assistance, a trained member of staff is able to build up a relationship with the complainant and then accompany them to meetings to offer support. In other Trusts, if appropriate, the chief executive may meet with the complainant to listen to their concerns. Wherever possible, complainants should be empowered to direct their own questions to staff members but some patients would prefer this to be done on their behalf.

If a number of staff are required to answer the complaint then the most productive way of having a meeting is for the complainant (together with a friend or advocate) to meet with a manager. The manager would then explain the procedure and invite the first member of staff to come in and answer the complainant's questions. The manager would summarise the responses at regular intervals and would also take notes. When the questions have been answered the manager would check to see if there are any further questions to be asked and summarise what has been said during the interview. When the staff member leaves they can contact the next member of staff and ask them to attend. Whilst waiting for the next member of staff the manager can discuss with the complainant what questions they would like to ask the next member of staff.

The meeting should be followed up with a written summary outlining the questions asked, the answers given and any other relevant information.

There is a danger that some complaints from patients with mental health problems could turn into serial complaints and therefore care should be taken to document carefully all meetings, telephone contacts and written correspondence.

Frequent complainers

Sometimes people with a personality disorder make a complaint and then come back with a different complaint either during the initial investigation or when a response has been sent out. Through this process they can then become dependent on the system. A suggestion in handling this type of complaint is for the complaints manager to talk to the clinical team caring for the patient to decide the best way forward, remembering that the complaint may or may not be caused by their illness. There may be a situation when the clinicians are trying to break the patient's dependency on a person or situation. What is subsequently happening is that the patient has transferred their dependency from their previous situation to the complaints process. In such a case the treatment of the patient with regard to the complaints department would become part of their care plan.

The legal status of complainants

A patient may be detained under the Mental Health Act:

- If it is in the interest of his or her own health
- If it is in the interest of his or her own safety
- For the protection of other people.

If the patient is not known to the services they may be admitted for assessment under Section 2 of the Mental Health Act. In order to carry this out the patient has to be seen by two medical practitioners (usually a psychiatrist and a general practitioner) and an approved social worker. If agreed between the three professionals concerned, the patient is subject to a 28-day assessment order in hospital.

If it is considered that a patient should be detained for treatment they may be subject to a 6-month treatment order under Section 3 of the Mental Health Act. This section of the Act can be renewed for a further period of 6 months and thereafter on a yearly basis as long as the patient continues to require treatment in hospital.

If the patient's condition is stabilised, they may be granted leave of absence, with conditions, from the hospital under Section 17 of the Act. For example, they may be allowed to go to the shops providing they return by a set time or be allowed home overnight or on extended leave, which may be for an indefinite period. Should they fail to comply with the conditions that have been laid down in writing, they can be recalled to the hospital. Refusal to take prescribed medication is not in itself grounds to recall a patient to hospital unless their mental health shows a marked deterioration.

In addition, patients may be admitted on a voluntary basis. In such instances patients would be able to take their own discharge if they so wished.

In some instances, patients making a complaint are, or have been, detained under the Mental Health Act. One reason they choose to complain may, for example, be because they object to being forced to have medication. It would not be possible to investigate a complaint of this nature if the treatment was given in accordance with the provisions of the Mental Health Act. In such circumstances the patient should be advised to apply to the Mental Health Review Tribunal and/or hospital managers for discharge from detention. If the patient complains that they were restrained inappropriately then the investigation must make sure that the control and restraint procedures were followed and clearly documented. If the procedures were followed, the patient should be informed that they were correct and documented in the care plan. However, an apology could be given for the distress they have suffered. If it was proved that the procedure was not followed, the disciplinary process would be invoked and police involvement may be appropriate if an assault had taken place.

Complaints records

Recording is particularly important with regard to mental health patients to indicate trends in both patient care and patient behaviour. Consideration should be given to recording all comments, compliments and complaints, whether they are received informally on the ward or in the form of a more formal written letter. Patients in long term care often make more observations than other patients and unless data is kept on the positive comments received, as well as the negative ones, a distorted picture may emerge.

Staff support

As with any staff working with complainants on a regular basis, staff dealing with mental health complaints may suffer stress due to the nature of the job. As was mentioned on page 34, senior managers need to consider how their staff should be supported and to make sure that the support is given in an appropriate way.

6

The Health Service Commissioner (the Ombudsman)

THE ROLE OF THE COMMISSIONER

The role of the Commissioner (or Ombudsman, as he is more generally known) is to investigate complaints about the National Health Service that have not been resolved locally. In law, there are separate Health Service Ombudsmen for England, Scotland and Wales but all three posts are held by the same person, currently Mr Michael Buckley, who has offices in London, Edinburgh and Cardiff.

The Ombudsman receives around 3000 complaints a year covering all sectors of the NHS. This figure, taken in conjunction with the number of patient contacts and the number of complaints received by Trusts and Health Authorities, implies that the vast majority of complaints are dealt with at the Local Resolution stage. As the Ombudsman is independent of the NHS and government, he is in a position to assist people who have suffered an injustice and to make sure that there are high standards of healthcare and public administration.

The Ombudsman:

- Can investigate a complaint only if it is put to him in writing (he cannot investigate oral complaints or start an investigation on his own initiative)
- Must tell the complainant why he has not investigated if he decides not to investigate a complaint
- Must give the person or organisation complained about the chance to comment before he starts an investigation
- Has the same powers as the courts to obtain papers, once he has begun an investigation
- Must send a report of his findings to the person who made the complaint, the person or body complained about and the appropriate Secretary of State, at the end of an investigation.

If a fault is found after an investigation the Ombudsman's report will contain recommendations to the health body to try to ensure that the problem does not reoccur. If the health body is unwilling to act on the recommendations of the Ombudsman, the Ombudsman can report to the Parliamentary Select Committee on Public Administration and, in turn, the Select Committee may invite senior officers from the health body concerned to give reasons for their actions. The Select Committee proceedings are usually held in public. More information about the work of the Select Committee is given at the end of this chapter.

AREAS THAT THE OMBUDSMAN CAN INVESTIGATE

In law, the Ombudsman's role is to investigate complaints alleging that hardship or injustice has been caused by:

- A failure in a service provided by an NHS body
- A failure of an NHS body to provide a service 'which it was a function of that body to provide'
- Maladministration by an NHS body.

In considering complaints about service failures the Ombudsman can examine the clinical judgement of doctors, nurses and other professionals if the events complained of happened after 31 March 1996.
   'Maladministration' can include:

- Avoidable delays
- Not following correct procedures
- Manner and attitude
- Not explaining decisions
- Not answering a complaint fully or promptly.

It can also include delay in dealing with, or a refusal to agree to, a request to disclose information that should be available under the Code of Practice on Openness in the NHS.

AREAS THAT THE OMBUDSMAN CANNOT INVESTIGATE

Areas that the Ombudsman cannot investigate include:

- Personnel issues including disciplinary matters
- Complaints from staff about their employment (but the Ombudsman can investigate complaints from members of staff about how a complaint against them has been handled by the health body)
- Commercial or contractual issues unless they relate to NHS contracts for patient services
- Properly made decisions, even if the complainant disagrees with them

- Services in a non-NHS hospital or nursing home unless the NHS pays for them
- Complaints involving the clinical judgement of a doctor, nurse or other professional where the events happened before 1 April 1996
- Complaints about government departments or local authority departments.

The Ombudsman might take up a complaint that has not been through all the stages of the NHS complaints procedure if, for example, there was evidence of unreasonable delay or maladministration in the complaint handling. Similarly, he might consider a complaint put to him more than a year after the events complained of if there had been delay in its consideration under the NHS complaints procedure.

HOW THE OMBUDSMAN DEALS WITH COMPLAINTS

On receipt, a complaint is first looked at by a team of officers who screen complaints to ensure that they cover areas within the Ombudsman's jurisdiction.

If the complainant has not provided all relevant papers the Ombudsman's office may ask the health body to do so. From the health body's perspective this is where a complaints log can be useful, as it will give the Ombudsman a clear overview of the documentation that has been enclosed, including details of how the complaint was handled and where and why the delays (if any) arose.

Once all the papers are to hand and it has been established that a complaint is within jurisdiction, the Ombudsman considers what, if any, action to take. He will not take action solely on the grounds that a complainant is dissatisfied with the service they received. Before an investigation is initiated the Ombudsman's officers have to be satisfied that the complainant may have suffered an injustice or hardship because the service has failed or because of maladministration.

If the complaint is concerned with clinical judgement the Ombudsman will take professional advice. The clinical advisors are asked to consider whether or not:

- There is evidence of fault in the management of patient care
- The complainant has been given an adequate explanation of the clinical issues
- The clinicians have acted reasonably.

If the health body has investigated the complaint, has acknowledged a fault, has given the complainant a clear and adequate explanation and apologies, has put in place systems to try to avoid the same thing happening again and has dealt properly with any request for an Independent

Review Panel, it is unlikely the Ombudsman will investigate. Instead, he would write to the complainant explaining why an investigation would be unlikely to achieve anything further. If it is clear that the health body is aware that a complaint has been put to the Ombudsman they will also be told of the decision not to investigate. The Ombudsman's office recognises that NHS bodies and others concerned with their work want as much information as possible and is looking at ways of providing more details of cases received and the progress of investigations and their outcomes with the aim of being as open as possible within the constraints of the legislation governing their work and the need to preserve individuals' confidentiality.

ACTION SHORT OF INVESTIGATION

With some complaints, the Ombudsman's office may either telephone or write to a health body and invite them to take further action. This could be for the convener to reconsider their action or for the chief executive to consider sending a fuller response. If the health body agrees then the complainant would be advised of the Ombudsman's action and the case would be closed (although the complainant would still have the right to approach the Ombudsman again if they remained dissatisfied after the health body has taken this further action).

In other cases, if a complaint was not handled correctly, but has not caused the complainant hardship or injustice, the Ombudsman would be unlikely to investigate but might write to the health body pointing out his concerns so that the health body could change procedures in order to prevent the situation happening again.

FORMAL INVESTIGATIONS

The Ombudsman will initiate a formal investigation if a complainant provides clear evidence to suggest that there may have been a service failure or maladministration, or if the papers provided by the complainant or the health body do not allow this to be ruled out on the balance of probability.

In these cases the Ombudsman's office will write to the health body informing them of the proposal to investigate and enclosing a Statement of Complaint, which sets the terms of reference for the proposed investigation. The health body will be asked to comment on the complaint and to provide relevant papers, usually including clinical records. They will also be asked to nominate a liaison officer to act as the point of contact for the Ombudsman's investigating officer.

What happens next will vary from case to case. It will often be possible for the Ombudsman to make findings and write a report without further investigation. This is particularly likely to be the case if the health body's response to the Statement of Complaint gives a clear and comprehensive account of events, which is supported by the clinical and other records, acknowledges shortcomings where appropriate and explains what action has been taken to prevent the problem happening again.

In other cases, limited further enquiries may be needed. For example, study of the papers may establish a need to look at relevant protocols or to discuss procedures with managers. In such cases the Ombudsman's investigating officer will ask the health body's liaison officer to provide copies of the relevant documents or to suggest who can be contacted, usually by telephone, to provide the necessary information.

In a number of cases, face-to-face interviews will be needed to gather evidence. The investigating officer will tell the liaison officer who will need to be interviewed and ask him or her to make the necessary arrangements.

The investigating officer conducts interviews in private. Where clinical issues are being considered, a professional assessor may accompany the investigating officer. The investigating officer will take notes and will generally check these with the person being interviewed during, or at the end of the interview. The person being interviewed is given the chance to comment on the written-up notes that the investigating officer will prepare after the interview. Anyone who is interviewed can be accompanied if they wish, but not by someone who will subsequently be interviewed. Interviews are not normally tape-recorded but, exceptionally, if both parties agree, a tape recording may be made. Persons interviewed are identified by job title, not name, in reports.

Once all the relevant evidence has been considered, the Ombudsman's office will produce a report setting out the facts of the case, findings and, where appropriate, recommendations. If clinical issues have been considered the advice given by any professional assessors appointed to advise on the case will be set out in the report or as an annex to it.

The report is sent in draft to the health body to establish whether any evidence given by their staff is inaccurately represented. If the complaint is upheld, the Ombudsman is likely to ask the health body to apologise to the complainant and may make recommendations, for example, to improve procedures. When the draft report is sent to the health body they are asked to agree to the apology and recommendations.

When the report is finalised it is sent to the complainant, the health body, any member of staff referred to specifically in the complaint and the relevant Secretary of State.

Periodically, the Ombudsman lays a selection of investigation reports before Parliament; the same reports are published and posted on the Ombudsman's website (www.ombudsman.org.uk). A health body will be given prior notice if the report of an investigation in which it was involved is to be published in this way. The complainant will also be notified.

Clinical Governance

THE SELECT COMMITTEE

The Parliamentary Select Committee on Public Administration may wish to take evidence from the senior staff of some of the health bodies involved in investigations where the report has been laid before Parliament. Generally, the cases the Select Committee considers are ones it feels to be particularly serious and/or raise issues of general interest, or where, in the Ombudsman's opinion, the health body has failed to co-operate with the investigation or act on any recommendations. Select Committee hearings are usually held in public and are sometimes broadcast. Transcripts of hearings are published.

Primary care complaints

SECTION CONTENTS

7

Can complaints be prevented?

WHAT IS A COMPLAINT?

When a group of practitioners or primary care staff meet together to discuss complaints someone will inevitably ask 'What is a complaint?' Probably the simplest definition is that a complaint occurs when a person makes an adverse comment about the practice. Using this definition, the vast majority of primary care complaints will fall into one of the following categories:

- Being unable to get through on the telephone
- Being kept waiting
- Patients coming late and being seen first
- The manner and attitude of the staff
- The practice not complying with their wishes.

The secret of preventing complaints is to try and anticipate problem areas and act first, rather than allowing a situation to develop that could give rise to a complaint. This can be done through auditing complaints received and looking for areas where systems could be changed or to identify problem areas.

Being unable to get through on the telephone

There are occasions when the telephone lines in a practice will be particularly busy and patients may have difficulty getting through; a typical time would be first thing on a Monday morning. However, a number of options can be considered if the phones are ringing constantly and no-one is available to answer them:

- Review the staffing rota – could the number of staff be increased during busy periods and decreased during quieter periods?
- Is an extra phone line required?
- Are other staff blocking the phones by making outgoing calls? Could they make these calls at another time or on a dedicated staff-only line?
- Are patients ringing for repeat prescriptions? Could they be encouraged to ring at a different time? Do all patients need to ring to request a repeat prescription or could some be generated automatically with a request at certain intervals for a review, for example, anyone on long-term, constant medication.
- Could patients be encouraged to ring at specific times for routine appointments, home visits, etc? Not all patients will comply but if 50% do it could well make a difference to the others who are trying to get through.
- Could one member of staff start earlier? For example, could the phone be answered from 8 a.m. on a Monday morning for the booking of urgent appointments and home visits?

If there has been a delay in answering the telephone, taking a few seconds to apologise for the delay could well prevent later complaints.

Being kept waiting

Patients who have arrived for a 9.00 a.m. appointment and are kept waiting without any explanation tend to get annoyed.

Patients may have been given correct appointment times but the practitioner may have been delayed in coming to the surgery or the surgery may be running late because one patient has taken longer than antici- pated. In this instance, the staff should inform patients about the delay as soon as they arrive, give the reason for it and apologise for the fact that the patient will be kept waiting. If the delay is lengthy (over an hour) the staff should consider the possibility that the patient could go away and return later if they wish or, in some instances, be offered another appointment. Staff need to remember that patients also have commit- ments, they may have to collect children from school, return to work, or return home to look after an elderly relative. The vast majority of patients will be happy to wait if the reason for any delay is explained as soon as they arrive.

People coming late and being seen first

Although staff easily understand the running of a surgery, patients do not always understand it. If a waiting area services several practitioners it is worth taking time to explain to patients who they will be seeing and that

primary care

there are several doctors in that morning. If there is a delay then the patients should be advised of the reason for the delay and be offered an apology.

The manner and attitude of the staff

Unfortunately, patients who are ill can sometimes behave in an inappropriate way. This can be due to anxiety about their condition, or that of a loved one, a lack of a firm diagnosis or a lack of understanding about what is wrong with them and the consequences that it may have for their future life. Staff dealing with patients should remain calm and professional at all times, however difficult that may be. If a patient does complain about the manner and attitude of staff an apology should be given, even if they in turn were rude. However, staff should not have to put up with repeated unacceptable behaviour from patients and a practitioner may need to become involved to point out that such behaviour is unacceptable.

The practice not complying with their wishes

Patients sometimes wish to see a specific practitioner, and to see them urgently. They do not appreciate that often the most popular practitioners have the most patients wishing to see them and therefore often have the longest waiting lists. It should be made clear why it is not possible for them to see that specific practitioner and an alternative appointment should be offered with someone else in the practice. Often, if the staff take time to explain the reasons why something is not possible, a patient will much more readily accept an alternative appointment or be prepared to wait, depending on the severity of their condition.

THE IMPORTANCE OF COMMUNICATION

Anyone who has had any experience of dealing with complaints will often say that the key to preventing complaints is communication. Communication may be verbal, non-verbal or written and may be staff-to-staff, staff-to-patient or relative, or relative-to-relative. Complaints are often initiated by what appears to be an insignificant incident, but one that is often the final straw in a series of 'little incidents'.

The following points should be considered when communicating with patients or relatives, they equally apply to all staff in the practice:

• Be on the same level as the person you are talking to (e.g. do not stand if they are sitting or vice versa)
• Try to maintain eye contact
• Speak slowly and pause to allow the person to ask questions

- Observe the person for signs that they do not understand what you are telling them
- Try to anticipate what the next question will be
- Do not rush the patient, especially if you are giving bad news.

Communication between staff members should be clear and records should be kept of any interaction between staff concerning the care of the patient or the information given to relatives.

Non-verbal communication is as important as verbal communication when talking with patients and relatives. It is possible to tell if someone is angry or upset by observing them carefully. Eye contact is very important and often indicates whether or not someone is being truthful; this applies to the person giving the information as well as to the person who is receiving it. By observing the person you are communicating with it is possible to tell how the information you are giving is being received, and to adjust it, if necessary. If, for example, it becomes apparent that the person does not understand what they are being told, or that they do not accept what they are being told, then presenting the information in a different way may help them to understand or accept the situation.

By closely observing patients in a waiting area it is possible to see if people are getting restless, especially if they have been waiting for some time or the room is very busy. Taking a few minutes to apologise for the delay and again, if possible, giving the reasons for it, can prevent complaints.

RECORD KEEPING

Accurate record keeping is key to the successful answering of a complaint. It is acknowledged that the staff are busy but records give a contemporaneous account of what actually happened. However, there is a tendency amongst some staff to think that if a situation is unchanged or that tests are negative there is no need to record the information.

If incidents happen in the waiting area it is worth keeping a record of what happened and who was involved. A book can be kept for the purpose as a central record is less likely to get lost than a loose piece of paper!

Telephone conversations should be recorded together with the date, time and the names of the parties involved in the conversation. This is especially important when talking to relatives who live some distance away, particularly if the patient is elderly or terminally ill. If a number of relatives are in contact with the practice, a record should be kept of what information has been given to each relative. Anyone investigating a complaint should be able to follow through exactly what has happened to the patient with regard to treatment and action as a result of tests. Dates and times of events become very important and, if they are present, can significantly speed up the time taken to investigate and therefore respond to a complainant. Experience shows that complainants who receive prompt and full responses are less likely to continue with their complaint.

POOR COMPLAINT HANDLING

If there is a clinical element to a complaint the practitioner concerned should always be involved in the response. There have been occasions when practice managers have felt that as the complaints lead they should handle all complaints but this is not the case in clinical complaints. The patient is entitled to an explanation of why a particular course of action was taken and only a practitioner can give the full explanation required in these cases.

A swift, full and accurate explanation will more often than not resolve a complaint but the converse can also occur. Therefore, it is not surprising to note that complainants who progress to an Independent Review Panel often complain about the way their complaint has been handled. There are occasions when a lot of work and effort is put into handling a complaint but it appears to be impossible to satisfy the complainant. Patients who may fall into this category are those who have suffered a sudden bereavement or have mental health problems. Conversely, it may be that although the staff have done a lot of work they have not actually addressed the complainant's concerns or they have used jargon or terminology that is not understood by the complainant.

PRACTICES FAILING TO ACT ON COMPLAINTS

Surveys over the years have shown that complainants say they do not wish the same thing to happen to anyone else and that this is the reason for their complaint. In view of this comment, practices should evaluate the complaints received and take action wherever possible to try to prevent a reoccurrence. Unfortunately, some practices that are very good at evaluating complaints fail to take this next step of changing practice.

One of the most constant themes that runs through complaints is the lack of communication. For example, an elderly woman was found to have a lump in her breast, which the doctor thought was a cyst but decided to refer to confirm the diagnosis. That evening she collapsed and was admitted to hospital where treatment was given for a deep vein thrombosis. Several weeks later her relative complained that she had not been referred urgently for a mammogram. The relative had not understood that although the breast needed attention, in view of the patient's age it was not judged to be life threatening, whereas the deep vein thrombosis was, and therefore had a much higher priority.

primary care

STAFF INVOLVEMENT

There will always be complaints in the NHS and it will not be possible to prevent all of them. However, staff can go a long way towards improving the way that services are delivered to patients. There should be a mechanism in place that enables staff to take note of, and act on, comments made by patients and relatives that result in action being taken. If someone says, 'I had difficulty with the steps' it is not sufficient to say, 'You could have used the other entrance where there is a ramp'. If the person had difficulty they probably did not know that there was a ramp, therefore, are extra signs needed on the steps to indicate where the ramp is?

New staff members are a source of valuable information as to how services can be improved. As they come from outside the practice they will notice areas of difficulty in the layout of notes or the design of clinics, forms, etc. Areas for potential improvement can therefore often be easily identified by interviewing new staff a few weeks after they have been in post.

ANALYSIS OF INDEPENDENT REVIEW PANELS

When looking at primary care Independent Review Panel reports it was noted that a large percentage involved the death of a patient. Further analysis indicated the following themes:

* poor communication
* poor record keeping
* missed or late diagnosis
* poor complaints handling.

There is therefore an implication that the way patients and relatives are handled before and after a bereavement is crucial to whether a complaint is received.

CONVEYING BAD NEWS

It is never easy to tell a person that a relative has died or that they are suffering from a life-threatening illness. When undertaking this task the following points may be helpful:

* The news should be given in person and not over the telephone
* The news should be given in private without interruptions from outside the room
* Tissues should be available
* A mirror and wash basin in the room allows people to freshen up if they have been emotionally upset.

Further guidance on how to conduct and record this kind of interview is given below:

Breaking bad news

- If the interview is to tell a patient bad news, ask them to bring a trusted friend or relative with them
- Check what the patient or relatives already know before giving further information
- Give the patient and their relative time to ask questions
- Remember that most patients do want to be told what is wrong with them
- Remember that a warning shot can be helpful (for example, I am afraid I have some bad news for you)
- If a person has died, refer to them by name
- After breaking the news watch and wait
- If the person becomes angry remember that it may be a displacement for other forms of distress and therefore the anger should be acknowledged and not met with anger
- Do not leave the patient and their relative(s) alone unless they request to be left alone, if so inform them of how to contact a member of staff
- Do not be ashamed about showing your feelings – people often appreciate knowing that the doctor or nurse cared
- If it is appropriate, leave the patient with a nurse and return after 30 minutes to answer questions
- The patient may cut short any explanation (e.g. I will leave all that to you, I will concentrate on getting better). If this happens, make a note in the records and return to the subject at the next consultation
- Consider giving only the most basic information at the first interview, follow-up with a more detailed explanation a few days later
- Make information available about where the family can get help and support, with the names and addresses of outside agencies including bereavement counselling and self-help groups
- Less educated patients and their relatives often ask for more information than people who have had more education, probably because they have less access to information or fewer skills to access it
- Use simple language; avoid euphemisms and medical jargon
- Probe to ensure that the person has understood; people do not always hear much of what is said after bad news has been delivered
- Make sure you have a clear method of recording what information each relative and patient has been told. In this way, doctors and nurses will be able to check and support the information given and it will be easier to judge who should receive further information and when and at what level it should be given.

primary care

What to record during the interview

- The key information the family has been given
- What written information they have been given
- If any medication has been prescribed
- If any tests have been organised
- If they have contact information about local support groups
- If they have a follow-up appointment for more information
- Who was present at the interview
- The time, place and duration of the interview
- Who is responsible for any further action required.

Discussions with bereavement care workers indicate that, ideally, a senior member of the medical staff should give bad news, as they would be in a position to answer any questions. It is helpful if a member of the nursing team can also be available to discuss any areas of concern that the patient or relatives may have if it is felt that this would be appropriate.

8

Local resolution

Local Resolution is the place where the vast majority of complaints are resolved. It is true that the quicker complaints are addressed and dealt with, the more likelihood there is for the complainant to be satisfied. If the practice staff are empowered to handle complaints, only the more complex issues may result in a written letter of complaint with the involvement of the practice complaints manager. As Chapter 7 dealt with the prevention of complaints, this chapter will concentrate on the efficient and effective handling of complaints.

RECEIVING THE INITIAL COMPLAINT

If a member of staff is approached by a patient or relative who is expressing dissatisfaction with the way a service is being offered, then, wherever possible, that member of staff should address the complaint. Bearing in mind the principles of the complaint system the person should be given a full explanation, an apology if appropriate and, wherever possible, steps should be put in place to try to prevent it happening again.

For example, if a patient complains that they are having to wait:

- explain why there is a delay
- apologise for the delay
- consider offering another appointment
- record the incident so that if this is a regular problem the information collected could be used as a basis to change systems. For example, longer appointment times may be required or surgeries may need to start later.

The above example may appear time consuming in a busy waiting area but in reality it will take very little time to address and the recording of the incident will demonstrate that action has been taken. One of the main problems with complaints is that if they eventually get to a convener there is sometimes a lack of supporting paper work. If there is no record of the conversation or action taken it is very difficult for the convener to make a decision.

Often, what appears on the surface to be a small complaint can grow out of all proportion in the later stages. The complainant feels frustrated that no one is taking them seriously and the staff feel that the complaint is taking up a disproportionate part of their time. Taking care in the early stages can often save a lot of time if the complaint continues through the process.

Initial checks and confidentiality

If the complainant is not the patient, be careful to make sure that patient confidentiality is not breached when answering the complaint. It is only possible to discuss the clinical aspects of a patient's care with a third party with the patient's consent. If a patient states that they do not wish other people to discuss their condition then that must be adhered to. In such a case it should be explained to the person complaining why it is not possible for you to answer the complaint and that the patient's wishes are paramount. Again, it is important that an outline of the conversation is recorded.

When to pass a complaint on

If a patient or relative comments to a junior member of staff, the member of staff should deal with the complaint only if they are capable of responding to if fully.

For example, if a patient complains that they have been waiting for a long time to see the practitioner, the member of staff involved should be able to say why they have been kept waiting and to apologise for the delay.

On the other hand, if a patient complains about the medical treatment they have received, the complaint must be passed on to the practitioner being complained about. The member of staff should explain to the patient why they are unable to respond and should also tell the patient the name of the person to whom they will be speaking about the complaint. They then need to pass the complaint on as quickly as possible to ensure that it is dealt with speedily.

THE COMPLAINTS MANAGER

Any written complaints are usually addressed to the complaints manager. On the receipt of a written complaint, the following questions should be asked before any action is taken.

primary care

- Is it appropriate for the NHS complaints procedure?
- Is consent required?
- Is access to medical records required?
- Is it a mixed sector complaint?
- Is the complaint out of time?
- Has disciplinary or legal action commenced?

Is it appropriate for the NHS complaints procedure?

The NHS complaints procedure is designed to deal with complaints about the provision of services by a practice for a particular patient.

Problems arise if issues not covered under the complaints procedure are dealt with under that procedure. Matters that are normally dealt with by other agencies, for example, noise from a Health Centre, which would be dealt with by the Environmental Health Department of the local authority, are therefore not covered. Complaints relating to accusations of sexual assault, assault or fraud may or may not be appropriate for the complaints procedure as they may be dealt with by either the Health Authority or the police, depending on the type of complaint. It is important to refer these complaints to the appropriate agency as soon as possible.

The complaints procedure does not cover medical care provided by a practitioner outside their NHS contract. However, NHS work undertaken in private hospitals but contracted for and paid for by the NHS does come under the complaints procedure providing that the contractual agreement covers the action taken in the case of a complaint arising from the treatment.

Is consent required?

If the complainant is not the patient then the patient's written consent will usually be required for the person to pursue the complaint on the patient's behalf. If the patient is a minor or unable to give consent then it is advisable to seek expert advice, as each case will rest on its own merit. If a child is in the care of an authority or voluntary organisation that organisation can bring a complaint on the child's behalf.

If a patient has died, a relative or an adult who had an interest in the patient's welfare may make the complaint.

Is access to medical records required?

If a patient is complaining about treatment they have received and, in order to investigate the complaint, their clinical records will have to be examined, technically their consent is not required. Unfortunately, patients do not always realise that non-medical staff will be looking at their records. The *primary care*

1

NHS Guidance states that the patients have a right to refuse to allow access to their medical records and, if this happens, it would not be possible to investigate the clinical aspect of the complaint. The question then needs to be asked that, if patients are not aware that their records need to be examined, how can they withhold consent? Consequently, it is advisable to inform patients that their records would be looked at and that their consent would be needed, this is especially important if the complainant is not the patient.

Is it a mixed sector complaint?

A complaint that covers primary and secondary care, or involves Social Services, is classed as a mixed sector complaint. The guiding principle is that a person needs to complain only once, and that it is up to the person receiving the complaint to pass the appropriate section of the complaint on to the other parties and to co-ordinate the responses.

Is the complaint out of time?

Complaints should be made within 6 months of the date the incident occurred, or within 6 months of the time that it came to the complainant's notice, providing no more than 12 months have elapsed from the original incident. If a complaint is received after the time specified it is up to the complaints manager to decide whether it would have been unreasonable for the complaint to be made earlier and that it is still possible to investigate the complaint properly.

It must be remembered that once a complaint has been accepted under the NHS complaints process then the complainant has the right to continue through the whole process. Staff should therefore ensure that it is possible to fully investigate a complaint before it is accepted. It is possible to tell people that a complaint is out of time and explain that it cannot be accepted under the complaints system but that the practice will endeavour to answer any questions. It would be necessary then to explain the limitations of any investigation and why it would not be possible to give a full explanation. For example, this could happen if a member of staff had left the practice.

Has disciplinary or legal action commenced?

If the complainant states that they intend to take legal action then the complaints process should stop. Some practices presume that a letter from a solicitor indicates that the complainant is taking legal action, this is not necessarily the case. The complaints manager should contact the solicitor concerned and ask if their client is taking legal action against the practice, this should clarify the situation.

ACKNOWLEDGEMENT LETTER

Any written complaint should be acknowledged by the practice within 2 working days of receipt of the complaint. This acknowledgement letter should inform the complainant, either in the body of the letter or by way of a complaints leaflet, of the following:

- The options open to the complainant under Local Resolution (written response, meeting)
- Where they can get help and advice (for example the CHC)
- When the complainant can expect a reply (within 10 working days)
- The options available if the complainant remains dissatisfied after Local Resolution
- Details of a contact person
- Details of the Health Service Commissioner.

THE INVESTIGATION

Once a complaint has been received and accepted then an investigation needs to be undertaken. This investigation is often done by the complaints manager or, if it is a clinical complaint, by the clinician complained against. One of the major problems associated with complaints investigation is the time involved in doing a thorough job but, as has been stated earlier, time taken at this stage can save a lot more time at a later date. In fact, a thorough investigation and response, handled in an open and honest way, will often resolve the complaint.

Problems arise when the people investigating the complaint do not speak to the staff directly involved in the complaint but instead say what they thought should have happened, forgetting that what may be a routine occurrence for them is often a once-in-a-lifetime experience for the patient or relative.

Conducting an investigation

The following steps should be taken when conducting an investigation:

- Collect the relevant papers
- Evaluate the letter of complaint
- Interview the staff concerned
- Investigate sources of support and advice
- Prepare a written response.

Collect the relevant papers

Before embarking on an investigation, collect together the letter of complaint, any other complaints correspondence, the appropriate section of the patient's records and any other supporting information. Examples could include the complaints book, appointment sheets, patient information sheets, consent forms, out of hours records.

Evaluate the letter of complaint

If possible, try to list the complaints as identified by the complainant. This will enable a check to be made to ensure that all the issues have been fully addressed. Identify which staff were involved with the patient at the time of the complaint and make arrangements to interview each of the staff involved.

Also try to identify what the person wants:

- Is it to improve the service for others?
- Has something gone wrong and they wish to know why it happened?
- Is it to understand what has happened to a relative?
- Could they be having difficulty in coming to terms with the loss of a loved one?

It is possible that the complaint identifies ways in which the service could be improved:

- Is it within your remit to bring about such improvements?
- Do more senior staff need to become involved?
- Could other areas benefit from the improvement?
- How could you disseminate any lessons learnt?

Interview the staff concerned

Many staff are deeply affected by complaints; it is not unusual for staff to recall complaints that happened many years previously. It is very easy, when reading one person's view of a situation, to presume that something very serious has happened, only to find that the picture changes completely when you hear the other side of the story. It is therefore vital to keep an open mind and to treat staff sensitively.

Interviews should be conducted in private and not in the middle of a reception area. Remind the staff that you are trying to establish what happened and wish to hear their version of events. Ask if they remember the patient and the incident referred to in the complaint and do not be surprised if they do not. Make sure that the appropriate records are available and allow the staff to remind themselves by reading the records. If the staff do not remember, and the information they give is from the records only, make sure that this is very clear in your report. Although the staff may not remember, the complainant will, and will notice any errors and draw conclusions, which may or may not be appropriate, from these errors.

Try to take each of the points raised in the complaint in turn. If information given is backed up by written records, say so, and where possible quote directly from the records. If there are omissions in the records it is important to say why the information was not recorded. Encourage the staff to make a written statement of their recollection of the events in question and ask them to date and sign it. They will find this useful if further questions arise.

Advise the staff where they can get help and support; sometimes staff become very upset and this can affect their work.

In clinical complaints, the practitioner complained about must always be involved in answering the complaint. There are occasions when a diagnosis is missed or it takes a long time to obtain a definitive diagnosis. Unfortunately, there is a perception amongst the general public that the medical professions can diagnose and cure all ills. If a diagnosis has been missed it is important to explain to the patient how the diagnosis would normally be arrived at. Then an explanation should be given as to why the normal diagnosis was not possible earlier. This could be because another condition was masking the symptoms or because no signs and symptoms were present. If it takes a long time to find out what is wrong with the patient they should be informed why it is taking so long and reassured that everything is being done to find out what is wrong with them.

Sources of support and advice

Advice and support when handling complex or difficult complaints can be obtained from the following people and organisations:

- The Local Representative Committee
- The Medical Defence Union
- The Medical Protection Society
- The Health Authority complaints manager.

The first three can help with the wording of letters and advise if there is a possibility of litigation. The Health Authority complaints manager can arrange for a lay conciliator to become involved.

Taking advice early on in the complaints process can ensure that letters are complete and correctly worded. A complaint that is handled correctly initially is much more likely to be resolved quickly and satisfactorily.

Prepare a written response

Depending on the practice policy, the response will either be sent from the complaints manager or the practitioner complained about. The most effective way of responding is to list all the areas of concern, use each one as a

primary care

heading and then provide the response under each heading. In this way it is very easy to check the reply, making sure that:

- All areas of concern have been covered
- All medical terms have been explained
- A lay person could understand the response
- Any background information that may help the complainant to understand what happened is supplied
- An apology is included, if it is appropriate
- If something has gone wrong, the steps taken to try and prevent it happening again have been included
- The information provided is accurate and complete
- If information is based on written records the records used are clearly identified
- If the staff do not remember an incident, it is stated that they do not remember and an explanation of what is normal practice is included
- The offer of a meeting is made, if appropriate
- Condolences are offered if the patient has died
- The complainant should be advised of their right to request an Independent Review Panel if they remain dissatisfied. Information should be given as to whom the request should be made and the 28-day time limit should be mentioned.

Informal meetings

Following the written response, a complainant may wish to speak to either the practice manager or the practitioner. The complaints manager will often be the person who arranges the meeting and attends to take notes of the proceedings. The factors listed below should be taken into account when a meeting is being organised:

- Who should attend
- The organisation of the room
- Paper work required
- Note taking
- Checking the notes
- The use of external clinicians
- The use of lay conciliators.

Who should attend

The complainant will wish to attend the meeting but it should be decided who can accompany them to the meeting. Often there are other relatives involved in the complaint and the complainant may wish to bring a CHC representative with them. On balance, it is often better to allow all the relatives who wish to attend to come with the complainant. It is often not clear from the correspondence what the main complaint is and in some instances the person writing the letter of complaint may be doing so on behalf of someone else.

If large numbers of relatives are attending it is better, if possible, to ask if they can agree that one person acts as the spokesperson for the group, although flexibility will be needed on behalf of the practice. A CHC representative often attends these meetings but, again, it is better if the complainant can be encouraged to ask their own questions rather than the CHC officer taking the lead. It must be remembered that it is the complainant's complaint and they are the only person who truly knows what their concerns are. In some instances it is only at a meeting that the true areas of concern emerge.

If the complaint involves a number of members of practice staff it is better that they do not all attend at the same time. It can be very intimidating for a complainant to walk into a room and be presented with a row of practitioners and nursing staff, along with the complaints manager. It also can give rise to comments that 'they were ganging up on me' or that the staff were 'sticking together'.

A more acceptable approach is for the complainant to initially meet the senior partner and the complaints manager, if they are taking the notes of the meeting. The other staff are then invited to attend one at a time, each answering the concerns raised by the complainant. When a member of staff has completed their discussions they then contact the next member of staff and ask them to attend the meeting. This approach gives the complainant time to gather their thoughts between seeing individual members of staff. It also means that the staff make much more effective use of their time.

The organisation of the room

Any meeting under Local Resolution should be as informal as possible. The use of low chairs and coffee tables may well be appropriate, as every effort should be made to ensure that the meeting does not become confrontational. The offer of tea or coffee and the availability of drinking water can also help. A box of tissues is advisable, especially in cases of bereavement – far better to have a box in the room than to have to go off and hunt for one if someone becomes upset. It is often more acceptable to the complainant for the meeting to take place in a non-patient area of the practice, especially in cases of bereavement. Again, it will depend on the nature of the complaint and the number of people attending.

If tables are used, try to make sure that everyone sits round the same table and, wherever possible, select a room that is neither too large nor too small. Use of an adjacent office where the CHC officer can talk to the complainant before and after the meeting is often appreciated. The officer can often provide feedback of the success of the meeting, although experience shows that it is usually very clear whether or not the meeting has satisfied the complainant.

Paperwork required

Wherever possible, make sure that the complaints file, the copy of the original letter of complaint and the written response is available at the meeting. If the response letter has listed the complaints, it makes the organisation of the meeting much easier if this is used as a basis for discussions. Prior to the meeting the complaints manager can discuss with the complainant which areas of their complaint they are still unhappy with and also which areas of the response they do not understand or do not agree with. This will then focus any discussions and make sure that the coi..plainant's concerns are answered fully.

The appropriate, original clinical records and any other supporting documentation should also be available at the meeting. This will enable the clinical staff to discuss the contents of the records with the complainant if required.

Note taking

It is important that a record is kept of the meeting. Although this does not need to be a verbatim report, it should say who attended the meeting and give the date and time. It is helpful if any explanations are noted under the appropriate areas of concern.

When taking notes of the meeting it should be remembered that if the complainant requests an Independent Review Panel they have to state what areas remain outstanding and why they remain dissatisfied. After taking clinical advice, the convener and the lay chair go through the correspondence (including the notes of any meetings) and decide whether or not a full explanation has been given. If the notes of the meeting simply state: 'The doctor answered the issues raised by the complainant' the convener and lay chair would not know what explanation was given or whether or not it was full. They would therefore have to decide whether to return the complaint to Local Resolution or grant an Independent Review Panel. If, on the other hand, the notes detailed what the doctor had said, they could decide that a full explanation had been given and nothing further could be added by granting an Independent Review Panel and therefore refuse the request.

Checking the notes

It is advisable for copies of the notes of the meeting to be sent to the staff involved for confirmation that they are an accurate record of the meeting.

primary care

Once the staff have checked the notes they can then be sent to the complainant with a request that they notify the practice if any corrections are needed. This ensures that the complainant has a record of the discussion that took place. Often, especially if they are upset, people do not remember all that was said at meetings. If they have the notes of the meeting they can re-read what was said and, in addition, more constructively discuss the content of the meeting with their relatives or the CHC. It also means that there is a full record on file for the convener, if necessary. If they are not sent the notes, the complainant could say that certain issues were not discussed. Asking them to agree the notes puts the practice in the position of demonstrating that the issues either had or had not been discussed.

The use of external clinicians

As the approach used for Local Resolution is up to the practice involved there may be instances when an external clinical opinion is brought in to help resolve a complaint. If, for example, a patient feels that the practice is covering up or that they are not providing all the information available, a review by an external person may help to resolve the complaint. The provision of a report by an independent practitioner, who provides an explanation for the clinical decisions taken and confirms that they were taken in line with current practice, may help to reassure the complainant. If, on the other hand, the independent clinician raises areas of concern then the practice has an opportunity to address these concerns and inform the complainant of the action that has been taken. It is not suggested that this is done as a matter of routine but there are occasions when this approach can provide a way through a particularly difficult complaint. This approach may be used as part of the lay conciliation process or perhaps the clinical governance lead from the Primary Care Group or Trust or another practitioner from the Primary Care Group or Trust could be asked to produce a report.

The use of lay conciliators

All Health Authorities have to appoint lay conciliators, who are widely used in primary care. There are several instances when the use of an independent conciliator can help to resolve a complaint. If the complainant refuses to meet with anyone in the practice and will not discuss their concerns, a conciliator can act as an 'honest broker'. They can meet with the complainant and then go and talk to the staff involved and provide a response. This is often useful if the complainant lives a long way away from the practice or has been removed from the practice list.

In cases of sudden bereavement, especially connected with the loss of a child or young person, the parents may direct their anger at the practitioner who looked after their child. They may feel that the practitioner was responsible for the death of their child and therefore will not believe any information that comes from the practice. If all parties are in agreement, a meeting with the parents and an independent clinician, facilitated by a lay conciliator, may provide the parents with some of the explanations and reassurances they need. To increase the likelihood of success the medical records should be available at the meeting and the clinician concerned will need to be familiar with the case.

A sudden death caused by septicaemia following meningitis would be an example of the type of case that may well benefit from this approach. The general public often does not realise that there are several types of meningitis. Instead, they want to know why a vaccination was not offered or, if their child had had a vaccination, why it did not work. They are unable to comprehend why their child died so quickly and may feel guilty that they did not act sooner. It is very difficult to provide answers to the above questions in writing. A discussion with explanations can often help, although it can never be said that the parents will be truly satisfied with any explanation given to them.

THE COMPLAINANT'S RIGHTS

The complainant has a right to request an Independent Review Panel within 28 days of the end of Local Resolution. It is therefore important that the final letter of Local Resolution advises the complainant of these rights.

The complaints manager or practitioner must send the final letter of Local Resolution although, if a conciliator has been involved, they may send the letter on behalf of the practice. One of the biggest problems is that it is very difficult to gauge which is the final letter. Local Resolution in primary care often goes through several stages, which may include:

- A written response
- A meeting with the staff concerned
- The use of lay conciliation.

If the complainant has received a complaints leaflet or the acknowledgement letter outlines the complaints process the original response letter could include a statement along the lines of:

I (the practitioner/complaints manager) have tried to give you a full response to your concerns. However, if you have further questions or remain dissatisfied, please contact (the complaints manager) within 28 days of this letter. He/she will explain the options open to you under the NHS complaints procedure.

The complainant should be given a contact address and telephone number. If they contact the practice they could be offered a further written response, a meeting or details of how to contact the convener, depending on the stage the complaint has reached.

Technically, once a complaint has been accepted under the complaints procedure if the 'last letter' of Local Resolution does not give the complainant the 28-day time limit then the complaint remains open. Therefore, if the complainant came back a year later they would not be 'out of time' as Local Resolution would be still in progress.

If the complainant wishes to request an Independent Review Panel they should be advised:

- How to contact the convener
- Of the 28-day time limit for making the request
- Where they can get help and assistance, for example the CHC
- To state what issues remain outstanding from Local Resolution
- To say why they remain dissatisfied.

primary care

9

Lay conciliation

WHAT IS CONCILIATION?

Health service conciliation is when an independent lay person communicates between a complainant and the complained against in order to enable both parties to have a full understanding of the areas of concern and to obtain a full explanation of why a particular course of action was undertaken.

HOW ARE CONCILIATORS APPOINTED?

Under the complaints legislation, all Health Authorities have to appoint at least one conciliator. This is a fixed-term appointment lasting for 1 year but it is subject to re-appointment. Certain groups of people may not be appointed as conciliators and these include people who are or have been registered as medical practitioners, dentists, pharmacists, opticians, members of a supplementary profession (for example physiotherapists, occupational therapists, radiographers, etc.) and nurses. In addition, the Health Authority has to consult with the Local Representative Committees before an appointment is made.

KEY AREAS FOR CONCILIATORS

Although the Health Authority appoints conciliators they work independently from it. Many have a contract or service agreement with the authority, which covers the issues shown below:

primary care

- Impartiality
- Confidentiality
- Data protection
- The return and storage of papers
- Professional advice
- Safety
- The NHS complaints procedure.

Impartiality

The role of the conciliator is to remain impartial throughout the process. Conciliation is not a judgemental process and therefore the conciliator should not offer an opinion as to whether or not a particular course of action was or was not appropriate. Any correspondence sent to one party should also be sent to the other party, for example letters summarising discussions at meetings. Both parties should always be treated equally.

Confidentiality

As the conciliator will have access to information about the patient, both from the patient themselves and from the practitioner, it is important that such information is not disclosed to an unauthorised third party. Consideration should be given to the storage and return of papers both during and at the close of conciliation. Care should be taken to make sure that, before any papers are sent, the conciliators do not know the parties involved so that they do not inadvertently see confidential information about a friend or colleague.

Data protection

Questions have been raised about whether or not conciliators should be registered under the Data Protection Act. Advice received from the Registrar indicates that this is not the case unless a conciliator keeps organised, identifiable patient files, or a database of complaints handled, at home. As information should be returned to the Health Authority, this situation should not arise.

The return and storage of papers

Care should be taken to ensure that papers are stored correctly and they should be returned to the Health Authority for storage at the end of the process. This can be done by placing the papers in a sealed envelope with details of both parties on the outside, along with the date and name of the conciliator. In this way, the Health Authority will not routinely see the information but it will be available if, for example, the convener asks for information concerning the conciliation process. Routine reports should not be made to the Health Authority about conciliation but anonymised information may be produced for statistical purposes. Such information could include the number of cases dealt with, the time taken to resolve the complaint and whether or not the complaint was satisfactorily resolved.

Professional advice

As conciliators are lay people they should have access to a professional advisor, who would normally be nominated by the Local Representative Committee. It is advisable for professional advice to be used in all clinical complaints as it can often assist the conciliator, and therefore the complainant, to understand why a particular course of action was taken or why it was not possible to make an earlier diagnosis. The clinical advisor can be used to:

- 'Translate' medical records and medical terminology into lay terms
- Explain the meaning of medical terms
- Give information about certain conditions, e.g. the different forms of meningitis
- Explain the difficulties in diagnosing certain conditions, e.g. the early onset of appendicitis, which can give the appearance of gastroenteritis
- Explain the typical signs and symptoms that are usual with certain diseases
- Explain the significance of test results
- Explain the progression of a specific disease
- Answer any specific clinical questions asked by the complainant.

Clinical advisors can be used either to provide information directly to the conciliator so that the conciliator has a full understanding before passing the information on to the complainant or to accompany conciliators to meetings with the complainant to offer independent explanations and answer questions directly. This is particularly useful if the complainant refuses to meet with the practitioner (and the practitioner agrees to the course of action, see page 78) in order to assist the complainant's understanding of why a particular course of action was, or was not taken.

Safety

The vast majority of complainants are reasonable people who genuinely feel that the system has let them down in some way. Unfortunately, there are some very rare occasions when complainants do not act rationally and may be very angry. It is important that the conciliator makes sure that they follow safe practice; consideration should be given to the following areas:

- Telephone number
- Address for correspondence
- Venue for meetings.

Telephone number

The conciliator should not release their home telephone number(s) to complainants as it may be very difficult to prevent a complainant from phoning at irregular or inconvenient times. If working from home, the conciliator can either use their own telephone and dial 141 to withhold their number or, if they have a dedicated fax line, use the fax phone, especially if it is unlisted.

Address for correspondence

Likewise, it is not advisable for the conciliator's home address to be used. The address for correspondence is usually either that of the Health Authority or a PO box that has been set up for use by the conciliator (and convener). Health Authorities that use the latter system have done so to demonstrate the 'independence' of the conciliator from the Health Authority. It is up to individual Authorities to decide which system they use.

Venue for meetings

Meetings can be held at a neutral venue, for example the Health Authority or CHC offices. This will depend on how convenient these buildings are for the complainant and the practitioner. It can be argued that meeting in a neutral venue is less confrontational.

Meetings are sometimes held in the practitioner's premises. This has the advantage that it is often easily accessible to the complainant, which can be an advantage in rural areas. In addition, supporting paperwork may be available, for example appointment books or nursing records.

It is not advisable to meet in the complainant's home as patients may be angry about what has happened to them and this can make the conciliator vulnerable to verbal or physical abuse. If a conciliator decides that it is appropriate to visit a complainant at their home then they should either be accompanied by a third party, for example a note taker, or they should inform a third party where and when they are making a visit and when the visit is over.

The NHS complaints procedure

As lay conciliation is part of the NHS complaints procedure, consideration should be given to the following aspects of the process:

- Conciliators are not permitted to report to the Health Authority about individual cases.
- Conciliation is part of Local Resolution and therefore has an advisory 'time limit' of 10 days. Whilst it is accepted that this is not always possible, one of the aims of conciliation should be to resolve complaints quickly.
- The final letter from Local Resolution must advise the complainant of their rights under the NHS complaints procedure. Conciliation should therefore be concluded with a letter, either from the practitioner or the conciliator on behalf of the practitioner, closing Local Resolution.
- It is permitted for the conciliator to discuss the case with the convener if a request has been made for an Independent Review Panel. The original NHS Guidance stated that this was not possible but further guidance issued under FHSL(96)45:ANNEX states that the convener may approach the conciliator in order to determine that everything that might have been done has been done in order to try to resolve a complaint.

WHEN IS CONCILIATION USED?

Conciliation is part of the Local Resolution process. In Trusts, due to their size and the number of patients seen over a year, the complaints managers tend to build up expertise in complaints handling. In primary care, although there has to be a person designated to take the lead in complaints, even in the larger practices there is not the volume of serious complaints to enable the manager to build up the expertise. The conciliator should have the expertise needed to handle the more difficult cases and also the time available to spend with both the complainant and the complained against in order to resolve the complaint.

Conciliation tends to be used in the more complex, often clinical cases or when there has been a bereavement or diagnosis of a terminal illness that has resulted in a complaint. In addition, it is used when the complainant has complained directly to the Health Authority and the staff feel that it would be inappropriate for the complainant to contact the practitioner directly. An example would be if parents felt that a practitioner contributed directly to the death of a child (even though the practitioner acted appropriately in the circumstances).

Either the complainant or the complained against can request the services of a conciliator, although both parties must agree to the procedure before conciliation can take place, this is usually done via the appropriate Health Authority.

CONCILIATION TECHNIQUES

There is no official guidance on the way conciliators should deal with cases and therefore the way they work is largely up to the individual conciliator.

Conciliation has therefore developed in different ways across the country. Since April 1996, when the existing complaints procedure began, conciliators have tended to become involved much later in the process, often when the parties have met or the complainant has already received a response from the practice. This is due to the change in policy, which introduced Local Resolution into the complaints process and, quite correctly, encouraged practitioners to answer complaints as soon as they arise.

As no two complaints are the same, conciliators need to be very flexible in the way that they work and be aware of a range of techniques that they can utilise in order to try to bring about a resolution of the complaints.

One or several of the following techniques may be used in a conciliation case.

- Telephone conversations
- One-to-one meetings
- Shuttle diplomacy
- A written response
- Meetings.

Telephone conversations

The conciliator may contact both parties by telephone to discuss the complaint. It is usual to telephone the complainant first so that the conciliator has a clear understanding of their concerns and what they wish to achieve by making the complaint. This initial conversation can often take over an hour as, although initially complainants will often say that they have nothing to add to their original letter, they will often then start to talk and elaborate. It is important that the conciliator allows the complainant time to talk as this in itself can often help to diffuse a situation. Many complainants say that just having someone neutral to talk to helps.

Eliciting what the complainant wishes to achieve through the conciliation process will help guide the conciliator as to the next course of action. The complainant may wish to have an apology and they may say that they do not wish the same thing to happen to someone else. Alternatively, they may wish to have the practitioner disciplined or 'struck off, or they may wish to have financial compensation. If a complainant raises a solution that is not possible it is important that this is addressed, as it would be unfair to continue and leave the complainant thinking that, for example, the practitioner will be disciplined. It may be possible to negotiate a reimbursement of money spent. For example, if a dental patient has had some dentures that do not fit, it may be possible to get the dentist to agree either to give the patient their money back so they can have the work redone elsewhere or to make another pair of dentures free of charge.

An advantage of using the telephone for the initial contact is that it can be very cost effective. The majority of complainants will have a telephone and it can enable the conciliator to make contact fairly quickly. It has been argued that some complainants are likely to feel able to discuss their concerns more freely on the telephone. One of the reasons given is that people always imagine someone nice when they are speaking to a stranger on the telephone!

When speaking to a practitioner on the telephone it is important that the conciliator does not indicate to the practice staff the reason for the call. Some practitioners do not discuss complaints with staff and occasionally the staff are not aware that a complaint has been received. Again, it is much more cost effective to telephone a practitioner and, for the less complicated complaints, may be all that is necessary to enable the conciliator to write to the complainant with the answers to the questions they have raised.

One-to-one meetings

It may be appropriate for the conciliator to meet with the complainant to discuss their complaint. This could be especially useful if the complainant is not on the telephone or if it is unclear from their letter what their specific complaint is. Wherever possible, such a meeting should take place on neutral ground, for example at the Health Authority or CHC offices. If the conciliator decides to visit the complainant's home then they should take care to ensure their own safety. The disadvantage of this approach is that it is often very time consuming and may add nothing extra to the original letter or the information gained through a telephone conversation.

A meeting with the practitioner may be appropriate, especially in more complex cases. This gives the conciliator an opportunity to negotiate a course of action, or to see records that support the practitioner's statements. These could include appointment books, test results or, if appropriate, the patient's records. If an error has occurred the practitioner could be encouraged to write and apologise and to explain what steps have been taken to prevent the error happening again. The conciliator can also encourage the practitioner to take advice from the appropriate Local Representative Committee, the Medical Defence Union or the Medical Protection Society, who will comment and advise on any letters written to the complainant. The disadvantages of this approach are that it can be time consuming and, unless it is very clearly explained to the complainant, it can be seen as the conciliator taking the side of the practitioner.

Shuttle diplomacy

In this technique the conciliator acts as a go-between for the two parties. This can either be done by telephone or by putting the parties in separate rooms with the conciliator moving between the rooms. The former technique can be effective but can also prolong the procedure, sometimes over weeks or months. As the spirit of the NHS complaints procedure is to resolve complaints as quickly as possible, the conciliator should ensure that they can contact the parties quickly and easily if this method is chosen. The latter course of action can be effective but it could be argued that, if both parties are in the same building at the same time, it is far better for them to meet if at all possible.

A written response

When producing a written response, the conciliator should bear in mind the aims of Local Resolution. Is it possible to negotiate an apology for the patient? For example:

Dr Smith has asked me to say that he/she is sorry that you were dissatisfied with the treatment you received.

If something has gone wrong, could the practice indicate what steps have been taken to try to prevent it from happening again? For example:

Dr Smith accepts that you were not telephoned with the results of your blood test, which was due to an administrative error. As a result of your letter the practice has reorganised the way in which blood test results are handled and hope that this reorganisation will prevent the same thing happening again.

Specific questions raised by the complainant can be put to the practitioner and the conciliator can write back to the complainant answering the specific points and giving the complainant a full explanation. If the complainant raises a more general question, for example, 'What are the signs and symptoms you would expect to see the week before someone had a heart attack?', as well as including the practitioner's answer the conciliator could ask the clinical advisor the same question and include their response in the letter. In this way, the complainant is getting an external explanation, and therefore a second opinion, which may help to resolve the complaint. This is very useful when a patient has died and the relatives have difficulty understanding why it was not possible to make an earlier diagnosis or predict that the death was going to happen.

As Local Resolution must be concluded with a written response, a decision will have to be made as to whether the conciliator can write the final letter on behalf of the practice or the practitioner should write the letter. It appears that it is more common for the conciliator to write if they have been involved, but this is not always the case. Whoever writes the letter, it must indicate the complainant's rights. As it is not known if it will be the final letter, paragraphs may be included which state, for example:

I have tried to give you as full an explanation as possible. If you have any further questions, or would like me to arrange a meeting, please contact ... at ... and she/he will arrange for me to contact you. If you are unhappy with any aspect of this investigation or wish to proceed to the next stage of the complaints procedure please contact … at … within 28 days from the date of this letter and he/she will explain the options open to you under the NHS complaints procedure.

If I have not heard from you within 28 days I will presume that you do not wish me to take any further action and therefore I shall arrange for your file to be closed.

If the letter contains clinical information the draft should be checked by the practitioner for clinical accuracy before it is sent out. For example, if the letter is written following a visit to the practice it may contain direct quotations from the medical records. For example:

You asked if the doctor took your father's blood pressure. In the medical records is an entry that states 'BP 120/80'. Dr Smith has informed me, and this has been confirmed by an independent medical advisor, that this blood pressure reading is normal.

In summary, a letter from a conciliator could contain some or all of the following points:

- Responses from the practitioner in answer to the complainant's specific questions
- Quotes from supporting documentation
- Independent clinical advice
- An apology from the practitioner
- If an error has occurred, what steps the practice is prepared to take to try and prevent it from happening again
- The offer of a meeting
- The offer to answer/discuss any further areas of concern
- The complainant's right under the NHS complaints procedure
- Condolences (if appropriate).

Meetings

Meetings can take place in a variety of ways; the venues for such meetings were discussed on page 72. When the meeting is between the complainant and the practitioner, with the conciliator facilitating, it is up to the conciliator to decide whether or not the parties can be accompanied, and by whom, but care should be taken to treat both parties equally. Allowing the complainant to bring a friend can be helpful as often another family member is involved in the complaint and it is useful for them to hear the explanations. Some CHCs wish to accompany complainants, which is useful providing the practitioner agrees. However, some practitioners see this as the patient being professionally represented and therefore wish to have someone from their Local Representative Committee with them, which can result in the meeting being much more formal.

primary care

What should be remembered is that it is the complainant's complaint and therefore, wherever possible, they should be empowered to ask the questions at the meeting. An effective technique is for the conciliator to meet with the complainant just before the meeting and to decide which questions they wish to ask and whether they wish to ask them themselves. If the meeting follows a written response it is often useful to use the letter as a basis for the discussions so that the complainant can identify which parts they do or do not agree with.

During the meeting the conciliator should summarise at regular intervals and check that the complainant fully understands the explanations given. If the questions are written down it is fairly easy for the conciliator to keep a record of the questions and the responses, so that the meeting can be followed-up with a letter summarising the content of the meeting, which is sent to both parties. The conciliator may have arranged for an independent practitioner to be present to answer more general clinical questions and to explain medical records or medical terminology. The independent practitioner could also be asked to check the final letter before it goes out to both parties to make sure that it is accurate, especially with regard to medical terminology and explanations.

If the complainant(s) do not wish to meet with the practitioner but wish to have an explanation, for example, about the course of a specific illness, it is possible, with the practitioner's consent and agreement, for the conciliator to meet with the complainant and an independent practitioner. The independent practitioner can then go through the records, explain what happened and answer specific questions about an illness. This can be particularly useful if a patient has died and the complainant blames the practitioner for the death even though there were no signs to indicate that this would be the course the illness would take. The meeting would follow a similar format to the meeting described above and would be concluded by a letter summarising the areas of discussion being sent to both parties.

INDEPENDENT REVIEW PANEL REQUESTS

If complainants have been provided with written explanations and written summaries of meetings they should be encouraged to include them with any request for an Independent Review Panel. The conciliator should also explain to the complainant that they would need to identify what issues remain outstanding from Local Resolution and why they remain dissatisfied before the convener will consider a request for a panel. It should also be explained that the complainant can get help and assistance from the local CHC and that the practitioner can get help from the Local Representative Committee, the Medical Protection Society or the Medical Defence Union.

SUPPORTING THE PARTICIPANTS

It may occasionally be necessary to advise the complainant or the practitioner where they can get support. If conciliators are aware of how to contact the local CHC, Bereavement Support Services, Counselling Services and The Samaritans, this information can be made available if appropriate and if requested by one of the parties. In an attempt to alleviate the stress encountered by professionals, some Local Representative Committees and Health Authorities provide access to confidential support for practitioners and, again, conciliators should be aware of how to access these services in case they are requested to do so by a practitioner.

primary care

10

The practitioner's role

When dealing with complainants, practitioners should remember that they are usually dealing with lay people and should therefore take care to avoid the use of medical jargon if at all possible. If jargon is unavoidable an attempt should be made to explain the terms used. Unfortunately, with the number of medical programmes in the media (both fact and fiction), the information available on the internet, the ability for patients to access their medical records and the volumes of written material available, the general public tend to use medical terms when they only partially understand the meaning of them. This can give the impression that they have a much greater understanding than they actually have. An example is the term 'distress'. To a lay person this can mean that someone is tearful or upset; to a practitioner it is often used as shorthand for respiratory distress, meaning difficulty in breathing.

Dealing correctly with complainants is time consuming but practitioners should remember that time taken early on can often save many hours of time later on by reducing the likelihood of the complaint moving on to the next stage of the procedure.

THE PRACTITIONER'S ROLE IN LOCAL RESOLUTION

Preventing complaints

All healthcare professionals should be aware of potential scenarios that may lead to a complaint and take steps to intervene. The following list gives examples but is by no means exhaustive.

primary care

• A surgery is running late – the receptionist or the practitioner goes into the waiting area, apologises for the delay and gives some indication of how long patients will have to wait.

• Relatives are demanding to see a senior member of staff and appear to have a number of 'trivial' questions – if possible arrange a meeting, in private. Consider having a nurse or the practice manager present to check understanding and to follow up with the relatives. Remember, their behaviour may be masking worries and concerns about the patient.

Oral complaints

Oral complaints should, if at all possible, be dealt with immediately. If a practitioner is asked to see either a patient or relative about a complaint then the sooner this happens, the more likely it is that the complaint will be resolved. It will be possible to answer the majority of oral complaints by explaining why a particular course of action has taken place and to answer questions fully and completely. Try to ensure that all questions have been answered and offer apologies if appropriate. Make sure that a record of the conversation is made including the date, time, who was present and the substance of the information given.

Responding to written complaints

In order to respond fully to written complaints, the practitioner will require the appropriate medical and/or nursing records. In order to provide a satisfactory response it is important that the following questions are answered:

• Is the response factually correct?
• Has any medical jargon been explained?
• Has a full explanation been given?
• If an error has occurred, has an apology been given?
• If an error has occurred, is there an explanation of the steps that will be taken to try to prevent it happening again?
• Have all the points in the letter been answered?

Experience has shown that complaints that progress to Independent Review Panels have done so because one or more of the above questions have not been addressed. Often, in order to save time, practitioners have said what they thought would have happened rather than what actually did happen, forgetting that to them the patient was one patient in a busy surgery but to the patient it may well have been a unique experience. If the practitioner is unable to recall a particular consultation it is far better to admit this and to say that the patient's medical records indicate that, for example, the blood pressure was taken and the patient's chest examined.

primary care

The response needs to be given in such a way that the complainant can fully understand the contents of the letter. Therefore abbreviations should be avoided wherever possible and medical terminology and test results should be explained.

A full explanation may well have to include information about why a certain procedure was not done or was not appropriate. If something has gone wrong, patients are entitled to an apology and the Medical Protection Society and the Medical Defence Union now encourage staff to apologise in such situations. From the complainant's perspective, many people simply 'do not wish it to happen to anyone else'. It is therefore important to explain if, and how, systems or procedures are being changed. Equally, if the complainant perceives that an error has been made but this error was unavoidable, then again a full explanation is required as to why it was unavoidable. For example, a patient attended with a sore throat and was sent home, septicaemia developed and the patient was rushed into hospital and later died. A full explanation would be needed as to why it was not possible to predict that septicaemia would develop.

Finally, it is also important to double-check that all the points raised in the initial letter have been answered. One approach is to use each complaint as a heading and then to answer each heading. This not only makes it easier to check that all the complaints have been covered but tends to focus the responses, making them easier to understand.

Participating in Local Resolution meetings

A meeting with a complainant provides an opportunity to give a verbal explanation and to answer as many underlying questions as possible. Although the emphasis is on informality it is advisable to have notes made of any meeting and to send a copy to the complainant for checking.

It is important to minimise the number of staff present at these meetings as a complainant can easily feel intimidated and the practice staff could well be accused of 'ganging up' against the complainant. If a number of staff are involved in a complaint, the easiest way of handling the large numbers is to see the staff one after another. Thus the first member of staff would see the patient and discuss their concerns. When they leave the room they contact the next person on the list, who then comes in. This process has the advantage that the complainant has an opportunity to gather their thoughts between seeing people; it is also a more efficient use of staff time.

Preparation prior to the meeting

It is important that the medical or nursing records are available and that the practitioner is familiar with the complaint and, if appropriate, has spoken directly to the staff involved prior to the meeting. It is important to be as factually accurate as possible and to check whether the staff recall either the patient or the incident that led up to the complaint.

At the meeting

Try to be honest – if you or your staff do not remember an incident, say so. It is then possible to go on to say what would usually happen in certain circumstances. You should be prepared to apologise if there were faults or omissions in the service that the patient received. It is important that jargon and abbreviations are not used and it can be helpful if there is a lay member of staff present (for example, the complaints manager or a lay conciliator) who can summarise at regular intervals and try to put any medical terminology into lay terms.

Allow the complainant to ask questions and listen carefully to the question being asked. It is better to ask for clarification before an answer is given than to answer the wrong question! By carefully watching the complainant it is usually possible to assess whether they have understood an explanation and it may be necessary to reword a response if you think the complainant has failed to understand the reply. In more complex medical situations it is sometimes helpful to use diagrams or anatomical models to aid understanding, rather than just words.

Before leaving the meeting, check that the complainant has no further questions. If there has been a bereavement an offer of condolences is always appreciated.

After the meeting

Check the record of the meeting carefully, to make sure that it is factually accurate. Ensure that a copy is sent to the complainant with a request that the practice be informed if there are any inaccuracies.

WORKING WITH LAY CONCILIATORS

A lay conciliator may become involved:

- If the complainant is not prepared to meet any of the staff in the practice
- With more complex clinical complaints; these often involve bereavement and the emotions associated with bereavement may be displayed at the meeting.

Methods of working with lay conciliators vary but it is usual for the independent practitioner to have a copy of the medical records and to advise the conciliator on the medical aspect of the case or to attend meetings with the conciliator. A meeting may be arranged with the complainant, the lay conciliator and the independent external practitioner. It is important that the original medical records are available and that the meeting is kept as informal as possible. Although the conciliator may ask questions on behalf of the complainant, it is more usual for the complainant to ask their own questions. The purpose of the meeting is to ensure that the complainant understands what happened and why a particular course of action was taken. It is useful to remember that the complainant may be feeling guilty for taking a particular course of action, for example, not contacting the doctor earlier, and may require reassurance that they acted appropriately under the circumstances.

It is usual for the conciliator to summarise at regular intervals, often putting words into lay terms. The conciliator may also ask for the meaning of medical terms to ensure the full understanding of the complainant.

As with the other Local Resolution meetings, it is important to check that the complainant has no further questions and to make sure that the summary of the meeting is checked carefully to ensure that it is factually accurate. The summary should then be included in the final response letter sent either by the practice or by the lay conciliator on behalf of the practice.

GIVING CLINICAL ADVICE AT THE CONVENING STAGE

If a request for an Independent Review Panel is made and all or part of the complaint is about clinical care, then clinical advice must be taken. The advice is taken by the convener and is passed on to the lay chair before the Convening Decision is made. Clinical advice is necessary because both the convener and the lay chair are lay people and therefore not necessarily familiar with medical terminology, the lay-out and contents of medical records and why a particular course of action has (or has not) been taken.

The clinical advisors are taken from a list supplied by the Local Representative Committee and arrangements are made with the local Regional Office for obtaining names of clinical advisors.

Documentation

The clinical advisor will require:

- A list of the clinical issues that the complainant feels are outstanding from Local Resolution
- Copies of any correspondence between the complainant and the practice
- The letters summarising any meetings that have taken place during Local Resolution
- The appropriate medical/nursing records.

primary care

Reviewing the records

It is not the function of the clinical advisor to comment on the appropriateness of the clinical action but to evaluate whether or not the aims of the complaints procedure have been met for each of the outstanding issues. For each of the outstanding clinical issues identified by the complainant, the clinical advisor should therefore assess whether:

- A full explanation has been given in a form that the complainant understands
- An apology has been given, if appropriate
- If something has gone wrong, an explanation has been given about the steps to be taken to try to prevent a reoccurrence
- All the clinical issues, as identified by the complainant, have been answered
- Any disputed clinical issues have been identified by the complainant.

It is helpful to both the convener and the lay chair that comments under each of the above headings can be written down, along with any suggestions for any further action that could be taken under Local Resolution.

For example, a particular treatment may have been given and the complainant says they feel that an alternative treatment should have been offered. If the correspondence only explained why the treatment was given, then a recommendation could be made that either a letter was written or a meeting was held to explain why the alternative treatment was not appropriate.

If, on the other hand, the advisor felt that the complainant was correct and that the explanation given was not in line with modern practice, they could recommend that the practitioner concerned reassess the treatment given and apologise to the complainant for not offering the alternative treatment.

Clinical advice is given in writing to make sure that both the lay chair and the convener receive the same clinical advice. In addition, the advice can be placed on file and will therefore form part of the audit trail if the complaints procedure is evaluated. If the convener refuses the request for the Independent Review, the substance of the clinical advice is passed on to the complainant and, again, it is helpful if reasons for the decisions are given. For example, where a particular point has been answered or to say that the treatment given was in line with current practice. In addition, the comments should be written in lay terms and any medical terminology or abbreviations should be explained.

When offering clinical advice, you may come across examples of clinical practice that give you cause for concern. As a practitioner, you have a duty of care to raise your concerns with the appropriate person but, if this is not an area that has been complained about, this should be done outside the complaints procedure.

Practitioners need to remember that, when giving clinical advice, they are looking only at the outstanding issues as identified by the complainant. It is therefore not necessary to review the whole of the treatment.

PROVIDING CLINICAL ASSESSMENT FOR THE INDEPENDENT REVIEW PANEL

The Department of Health has compiled a list of people who are willing to act as clinical assessors and this list is consulted when a request is made by a Health Authority for clinical assessors to advise the lay Independent Review Panel members. Clinical assessors are appointed from outside the practice area. There is a minimum of two assessors for an Independent Review Panel with a clinical element.

When appointed, the clinical assessors should receive the following information:

• Details of the parties involved in the complaint. The assessors should make sure that they do not know either of the parties before agreeing to accept the appointment.
• A letter of appointment, which should include indemnity cover for the assessor whilst they are working on the complaint.
• A claim form for the fees.
• The terms of reference for the Independent Review Panel. These will limit the workings of the panel and indicate the areas on which the assessors should concentrate when writing their reports and questioning the parties.
• Copies of the correspondence between the complainant and the practice, including the letters summarising any meetings that have taken place.
• Copies of the relevant medical/nursing records.
• Any additional documentation, for example post-mortem reports, death certificates.
• The names and position of the other assessor(s) and the panel members.
• A contact name and telephone number of the person at the Health Authority who is co-ordinating the review.

The preliminary report

After receiving the papers, each clinical assessor should review the papers and evaluate whether:

• Any additional papers will be required
• It will be necessary to physically examine the patient prior to the Independent Review Panel

primary care

- Any equipment will be required on the day of the panel, for example, X-ray viewing boxes
- They would like to interview any additional members of staff at the Independent Review Panel.

Increasingly, panels are asking clinical assessors to produce a preliminary report, which is made available only to the panel, prior to the Independent Review Panel. This report should be based on the written information only. These preliminary reports help the panel to understand the clinical aspects of the case, indicate whether there are any differences of clinical practice between the assessors and enable the panel members to identify areas of the complaint that may require clarification.

The suggested content of the preliminary report would be a summary of the clinical aspects of the case, bearing in mind the terms of reference. The findings of the assessor, and any recommendations, should appear under each term of reference. Recommendations should be based on how to improve the effectiveness and efficiency of the service provided for future patients. It is important that the recommendations do not suggest disciplinary action as it is clearly indicated in the underpinning legislation that the panel cannot make recommendations about disciplinary action. As the report will be read by lay people, it should concentrate on the clinical aspects of the terms of reference. Wherever possible, abbreviations should be avoided and any medical terms explained. It is also helpful to the panel to explain why a particular course of action or treatment was, or was not, taken.

The preliminary report should be sent to the Health Authority for circulation to the panel members in advance of the meeting. This enables the members to read the report and formulate any questions that they may wish to ask on its contents.

At the Independent Review Panel

It is becoming increasingly common for the panel members and the clinical assessors to meet for about half an hour immediately prior to the Independent Review Panel. This enables the panel members to meet each other and to question the clinical assessors on any areas of the complaint they do not understand and to clarify issues that may have arisen from the reports. In addition, the lay chair is able to indicate which areas of the complaint the panel members and the clinical assessors should lead on and establish the order of the questioning and the method of working of the panel.

During the Independent Review Panel hearing it is usual for the clinical assessors to take the lead on the clinical aspects of the complaint both when the complainant and the complained against are being interviewed. Many lay chairs allow the complainant to ask the clinical assessors for explanations and clarification about certain aspects of the complaint; the

primary care

panel members and the lay chair can also ask the clinical assessors to explain clinical issues. Care must be taken to ensure that both parties are treated equally and fairly.

A trend is now emerging that, immediately after the Independent Review Panel, the panel members and the clinical assessors meet to decide the findings of fact and any recommendations that the panel may wish to make. This course of action makes the final report truly a panel report and not just the view of one individual. If the clinical assessors have produced preliminary reports it is sometimes possible for them to dictate their final report, which can either be a joint report or individual reports. The final report(s) will be appended to the panel's report and will therefore be seen by the complainant. The report(s) should therefore be checked again to ensure that appropriate language is used and that they do not contain information that could cause 'serious harm' to the patient. It is helpful to the panel if the assessor's reports are produced as quickly as possible following the Independent Review Panel, as it is not possible to finalise the panel's report until the assessor's reports have been received.

STAFF SUPPORT

Many practitioners are adversely affected by being on the receiving end of a complaint; it is not unusual for them to report stress and sleepless nights. However, many try to cover up their stress, which may show in the form of aggression or simply ignoring the complaint and hoping it will go away. In extreme cases, staff have taken time off sick when the effect of a complaint has added to the stress of a busy workload. The Local Representative Committee, Occupational Health, the Medical Defence Union and the Medical Protection Society all offer help and support, and information on how they can be contacted should be freely available to all staff. People do not forget if a complaint has been made against them and many can recall the incident in vivid detail many years after the original complaint has been dealt with.

Senior staff and managers should be aware of the effects complaints have on staff and should be prepared to support them and to advise on external sources of support if appropriate.

Complaints should always, initially, be discussed with individual staff members in private and care should be taken to listen to the member of staff's side of events before any judgements are made. The listening time given to staff at this stage can be invaluable in supporting them during this period. If junior partners have to attend meetings, a more senior member of staff should take time to explain the process fully and advise where they can get help and advice. The Local Representative Committee, the Medical Protection Society and the Medical Defence Union are available to give support and may accompany practitioners to a hearing if required.

11

The Health Service Commissioner in primary care

Each year, the Health Service Commissioner (the Ombudsman) produces an annual report commenting on the previous year's work and outlining lessons that can be learned through the complaints procedure. He indicates areas of concern and potential areas where complaints can be prevented. In addition, he publishes information and reports on cases that have been investigated, usually at quarterly intervals. The reports are also available on the internet and are therefore easily accessible. This chapter will consider the key messages coming out of the Ombudsman's reports, with regard to primary care and Health Authority complaints.

The theme running through the reports is that the Ombudsman has to decide if a practitioner's actions have been fair, reasonable and consistent with those of the practitioner's peers. At the time of writing (June 2000), the Ombudsman is unable to investigate practitioners who have retired or who have ceased to work for the NHS. However, a Private Members Bill currently going through Parliament would permit such investigations.

COMPLAINTS HANDLING

The principle behind the complaints procedure is that complaints should be handled as quickly as possible and the professional bodies have issued guidance to this effect. However, the Ombudsman has identified that, in spite of the guidance, some practices delay in responding to complaints and others do not respond in a helpful or constructive way. There is apparently evidence to show that some practices fail to inform complainants of their right to request an Independent Review Panel, or how they should go about making the request and to whom it should be made. Also, some practices close complaints too early, before giving complainants the opportunity to have a meeting or before answering further questions that have been raised in the initial response.

OUT-OF-HOURS TREATMENT

General practitioners are responsible for making arrangements for out-of-hours treatment for their patients. In the year 1998–9, the Ombudsman held the deputising services, in addition to the practitioners, accountable for their actions in two cases.

THE NAMING OF GENERAL PRACTITIONERS

Removal of patients

Although, technically, a general practitioner does not have to tell a patient why they have been removed from the list, it is considered good practice to do so. If patients are not informed as to why they have been removed from a list they will be unable to change or modify their behaviour if this was the reason for their removal. If the patient complains about being taken off a practitioner's list then they are entitled, under the NHS complaints procedure, to have their complaint investigated and answered.

The Ombudsman has said that he will name general practitioners who take patients from their list solely because they have complained, as he does not consider this action to be fair and reasonable.

Rejecting recommendations

The Ombudsman will not normally name general practitioners in reports, only the Health Authority or Health Board area in which they practice. If the Ombudsman investigates a complaint against a general practitioner and makes recommendations in the report, the practitioner will be invited to act on the recommendations. If the practitioner rejects the recommendations made by the Ombudsman then he has said that he will name the practitioner concerned.

OTHER PRACTITIONERS

Although the majority of complaints received by the Ombudsman are about the care and treatment given by general practitioners, complaints are received about other primary care professionals.

Dentists

The key message about the dental service concerns communication with patients. It is accepted that most dentists do private and NHS work and, when offering private treatment to NHS patients, it is important that the dentist gives patients a clear explanation about the alternative NHS treatment and the cost of such treatment.

Pharmacists

The key message about the pharmaceutical services concerns the incorrect dispensing of medication. If it is found that a patient has been given the incorrect drug or an incorrect dosage then it is important that the patient's own general practitioner is informed about what has happened so that they can act accordingly.

THE HEALTH AUTHORITY
Complaints about Local Resolution

If a complainant writes to the chief executive of the Health Authority complaining about the way a practitioner has dealt with a complaint under Local Resolution, the complaint should be referred to the convener. The convener should then treat the letter as if it were a request for an Independent Review Panel.

Complaints about an Independent Review Panel

If a practitioner is dissatisfied with the way that an Independent Review Panel was run they should write to the Ombudsman, who will then decide whether or not to investigate their complaint.

The Health Authority's role

The Convening Decision

If a complainant is dissatisfied with the outcome of Local Resolution they have 28 days to write to the Health Authority's convener to request an Independent Review Panel. The convener, in consultation with an independent lay chair, will decide whether to allow the request. In the case of clinical complaints the convener will need to take advice from a practitioner who has been nominated as a clinical advisor by the Local Representative Committee and allocated by the appropriate Regional Office.

THE COMPLAINTS MANAGER

The complaints manager is responsible for providing the administrative support for the Convening Decision. All parties will require a copy of all correspondence between the complainant and the practitioner, along with the minutes of any meetings that have taken place and the file notes of any conversations. It is helpful to all concerned if the papers are put in date order and are numbered before being photocopied. In addition, the clinical advisor will require copies of the relevant medical records.

The complaints manager will also be responsible for making sure that:

- The initial checks and associated paper work have been completed
- Acknowledgement letters are sent out (the time limit is 2 days for the acknowledgement by the convener)
- The identification and the appointment of the lay chair takes place at the earliest possible stage
- The outstanding issues have been identified
- The time limit of 10 days for the Convening Decision is being adhered to
- All parties are informed of the reason for the delay if the time limits are not going to be met
- The papers are returned at the end of the Convening Decision and are stored separately from the patient records
- Expenses forms are completed and processed promptly.

THE INITIAL CHECKS

Knowledge of the parties

Before the papers are sent to the convener or other members of the team it is important to check that the complainant is not known to any of the people involved in the Convening Decision. It is not acceptable to send out the papers and then ask the question.

Time limits

As the complainant should make the request for an Independent Review Panel within 28 calendar days of the final letter of Local Resolution, a check should be made on the dates of both letters. If the request is made outside the 28-day limit, it is up to the convener to decide whether or not it would have been unreasonable for the complainant to make the request within the time scales. It is possible for the time scales to be extended, for example, if the complainant has been ill and therefore unable to meet the 28-day deadline. In addition, the convener should decide whether or not it would still be possible to investigate the complaint properly.

One problem that may be encountered is that complainants have not received a final letter. In other words, the practice has not advised them that they have 28 days to request an Independent Review Panel. Technically, if the complainant has not received a letter giving this information then the complaint is still in Local Resolution and therefore cannot be judged to be out of time.

Outstanding issues

It is very clear in the directions that the complainant needs to:

- Identify, in writing, the issues that remain outstanding from Local Resolution
- Say why they remain dissatisfied.

If the initial request from the complainant does not state which issues remain outstanding and why they remain dissatisfied the complaints manager may write to the complainant advising them that these statements are necessary in order for the convener to consider the request. It is helpful if the complainant can be advised of the names, addresses and telephone numbers of people who could assist them, for example the local CHC or the Citizens' Advice Bureau. In addition, the complainant should be advised of a date by which the Health Authority would expect to hear from them, as one of the principles behind the complaints procedure is that complaints should be dealt with as quickly as possible. A reasonable time to expect a response would be in the order of 10 working days.

If the complainant writes back and still fails to identify the outstanding issues and their reasons for remaining dissatisfied it is possible for the convener or a member of staff to list all the issues in a letter, which is sent to the complainant with a request that they confirm that all the issues have been covered. It will make the convener's role much easier if, when writing this letter, the issues are presented in date order and are numbered. This ensures that all issues are covered in any subsequent correspondence. Again, it is helpful if the complainant can be advised of a date when the Health Authority would expect to hear from them.

THE APPOINTMENT OF PARTIES

The convener

The number of conveners appointed by a Health Authority will depend on the size of the Health Authority. Every Health Authority must appoint one non-executive to take on the role of the convener but additional associate conveners may also be appointed. If the convener is a non-executive director they do not receive extra payment for their role as convener and are indemnified for this role in the same way that they are indemnified for carrying out their role as non-executive director.

Associate conveners can be reimbursed sessional fees at the rate determined by the Health Authority, in additional to travel and out-of-pocket expenses. Associate conveners should also be indemnified by the Health Authority for their work.

The appropriate Regional Office should be advised of the appointment of a new convener.

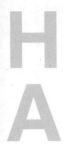

Health Authority

The lay chair

The appropriate Regional Office is responsible for recruiting and training the lay chairs. These are people who are not involved with the Health Authority and who provide the independent element to the Convening Decision process.

When a request for an Independent Review Panel is received, a request is made to the Regional Office for a lay chair. The regional officers nominate a lay chair and in doing so try to ensure that, wherever possible, the lay chair has not been involved with a previous Independent Review request at that Health Authority. This is done in order to ensure that the independence of the lay chair is maintained and that the lay chair does not get too involved with a Health Authority.

Once the name of the lay chair is known, and after the check is made to ensure that the lay chair does not know the parties concerned, a formal letter of appointment is sent out from the Health Authority.

As from this point the lay chair is working for the Health Authority, the letter of appointment should include the following:

- A confidentiality statement
- Confirmation that indemnity cover is provided
- Details of travel, subsistence and financial loss allowance payable
- Details of how to claim for incidental expenses, such as postage and telephone costs
- Instructions about the return of papers
- Details of how to contact the convener
- A contact name at the Health Authority with an address, telephone and fax numbers along with an e-mail address.

A confidentiality statement

The lay chair will see the letters and notes of any meetings that have taken place in the course of the investigation of the complaint. Some of the papers may contain details about the patient's medical condition. With the advent of the Caldicott Guardians, a very high level of importance is attached to confidentiality and Health Authorities have a duty of care to ensure that any information concerning patients is handled correctly.

To ensure that people act appropriately they should be reminded of the importance of:

- Confidentiality
- The correct storage of papers
- Not discussing the complaint with any third party in any way that identifies the complainant.

Confirmation that indemnity cover is provided

As the lay chair will be working for the Health Authority when they take part in the Convening Decision, they should be indemnified by the Health Authority for their work. HSC 1998/010 *Personal liability of non-executive directors of NHS Trusts, non-executive members of Health Authorities and non-executives of Special Health Authorities* and HSG (99) 104 *Personal liability of non-executives: Amendment of indemnity*, give the framework for this indemnity cover. The wording recommended is as follows:

A chairman or non-executive member or director who has acted honestly and in good faith will not have to meet out of his or her own personal resources any personal civil liability which is incurred in the execution or purported execution of his or her board function, save where the person has acted recklessly.

It is important that letters of indemnity are signed by the chief executive of the Health Authority.

Travel, subsistence and financial loss allowance payable

The Department of Health produces guidance on these rates. Lay chairs cannot be paid for the work that they undertake but they are able to claim demonstrable loss of earnings. Therefore, if a lay chair took time off from work and their salary was reduced as a result, they could claim back that loss. There is a problem around self-employed people as the payment is for actual, rather than potential, loss of earnings. It is advisable that the Health Authority formulates a policy for payment, possibly including a maximum daily rate that they are prepared to reimburse.

How to claim for incidental expenses

The Health Authority should be prepared to reimburse the cost of postage, phone calls and travel. The lay chair should be informed of the rates the Authority is prepared to pay and should be sent a claim form with information concerning when the form should be returned and to whom.

Instructions about the return of papers

As has already been mentioned, the Health Authority has a duty of care to make sure that patient information does not get into the public domain. The Department of Health has stated that complaint papers should be stored for the same length of time as patient's records. Thus, if all records are returned to the Health Authority on the completion of the Convening Decision, a full set of records can be stored. Personal notes made by the lay chair can be placed in an envelope and stored with the records so that they can be retrieved at a later date if required. It is not satisfactory for the lay chair, or anyone else involved in the process, to destroy any of the records themselves – how would the Health Authority know they had been destroyed correctly? In one instance, a lay chair said they always burnt papers, which on the face of it sounded appropriate. However, on further questioning it turned out that what they actually did was place the papers in a plastic sack and take them to the local refuse tip for incineration. It had not occurred to them that this course of action made it possible for those documents to be accessed by a third person prior to incineration.

Contact details

It can save much time and effort if full contact details are supplied at the beginning of the process. The use of e-mail is increasing and many lay chairs have fax facilities available to them. Having a named person who can be contacted at the Health Authority ensures that the process can be handled efficiently, hopefully within the 10 working days allocated to the Convening Decision.

The clinical advisors

If the complaint contains a clinical element then the convener must take clinical advice. The Local Representative Committees have been asked to supply the Regional Office with names of practitioners who are prepared to give such advice. Therefore, if a complaint concerns a general practitioner then the name of a general practitioner to act as an independent clinical advisor will be required from the regional list. If the complaint also involves the practice nurse then a nursing advisor will also be required to advise on that aspect of the complaint.

THE PRINCIPLES BEHIND THE CONVENING DECISION

The aim of the Convening Decision is for the convener, in conjunction with the lay chair, to evaluate whether or not the aims of the complaints procedure have been met. Namely:

- Has a full and complete explanation of what happened, and why, been given in terminology that the complainant can understand?
- Has an apology been given if there was an error or omission on behalf of the practice staff?
- If there was an error or omission, has information been given about the action that the practice has taken, or is proposing to take, to try to prevent it happening again?

Health Authority

Health Authority

In addition, can any further information be given to the complainant to help resolve the complaint?

Independence versus impartiality

One of the criticisms levied at the Convening Decision is that if the convener is a non-executive member of the Health Authority, how can they be independent? It is important to realise that the convener is not independent of the Health Authority – they cannot be, as they are responsible for the actions of the Health Authority. What the convener is able to be is impartial. They should not 'take sides', nor should they write as if they are acting on behalf of the Health Authority. They should try to take as structured an approach as possible and should be able to demonstrate their impartiality by the way they handle the decision-making process.

On the other hand, the lay chair *is* independent from the Health Authority. As has already been mentioned, the Regional Office tries to allocate a different lay chair for each Independent Review Panel request to maintain the independence.

Misunderstandings can arise from the language and terminology used in some complaints leaflets and correspondence. When checking literature it may be useful to bear in mind the following points:

- It is *the convener*, not the independent convener
- The *convener is impartial,* not independent
- It is *the independent lay chair*
- The convener obtains *independent* clinical advice.

What is being evaluated?

The convener, the lay chair and the clinical advisor have copies of:

- The outstanding issues as identified by, or approved by, the complainant
- All correspondence between the complainant and the practice
- Notes of meetings that have taken place during Local Resolution; these should have been agreed by the complainant.

In addition, the clinical advisor has copies of the appropriate medical, dental, pharmaceutical, optical or nursing records.

The convener, the lay chair and the clinical advisor look at each of the outstanding issues in turn. Their role is to evaluate whether the aims of the complaints procedure have been met for each of the issues that remain outstanding. If the aims have not been met they need to decide whether more could be done at Local Resolution or if the only way to satisfy the complainant is to convene an Independent Review Panel.

Health Authority

Therefore, the purpose of the Convening Decision is not to pass judgement on the treatment but to evaluate the Local Resolution process. If an error has been made, has been acknowledged by the practice, an apology given and the steps that have been taken to try to prevent it happening again outlined, then there is no further action that can be taken and any request for an Independent Review Panel should be refused.

AN OVERVIEW OF THE CONVENING DECISION

The role of the convener and the lay chair is to review the correspondence and file notes from Local Resolution and decide whether the aims of the complaints process have been met for each of the outstanding issues outlined by the complainant.

Should the parties be interviewed?

The guidance document produced by the NHS Executive suggests that the convener and lay chair may wish to interview the parties involved. However, in subsequent Health Service Commissioner reports the Ombudsman has criticised conveners for investigating complaints. Over the years it has become clear that, although technically the convener and the lay chair may talk to the complainant, this should be done only in exceptional circumstances. If the complainant is unable to state what issues are outstanding it is better to advise them where they can get assistance (for example, from the CHC), than to involve the convener. Unfortunately, it is very difficult for the convener to avoid being drawn into a complaint if they have direct contact with a complainant. The convener may be asked:

- Do you think I have grounds for complaint?
- Don't you think I should have had the tests?
- Have you had many complaints about X?
- Lots of people I know have had the same complaint about X; don't you find he/she is always rude to patients?

Answering any of the above questions will draw the convener into the complaint and, potentially, place them in the position of either being accused of investigating the complaint or of not treating both parties equally. It could also be argued that, if the convener talks to one of the parties, they should also talk to the other party and thus they become even more involved.

Some conveners (and lay chairs) have said that if only they could talk to the parties they could resolve the complaint. This may well be true but it is not their role; it *is* the role of the practice staff, the Health Authority conciliator in Local Resolution or the Independent Review Panel. On balance, it would therefore be advisable for conveners not to have direct contact with any of the parties involved in the complaint.

Taking clinical advice

When the complaints procedure first came into being, many conveners met with the clinical advisors and discussed the complaint with them. The conveners argued that they needed to see the clinical records and discuss the complaint in order to understand it. By taking this line they showed that they had misunderstood their role. If, after reading the letters of explanation sent out by the practice to the patient and looking at the notes of meetings where explanations had been given, they failed to understand the explanation of the complaint, then it would be reasonable to assume that the complainant would also fail to understand it! This would probably explain why the complainant had requested an Independent Review Panel. The convener's role would then be to decide where best to get the full explanation required – either in further Local Resolution or by convening an Independent Review Panel.

Clinical advisors received very little training when the complaints procedure first came into being. As a result, many felt that their role was to review the whole case and comment on whether or not the action taken was appropriate. This is not their role under the current complaints procedure. A convener who asks specific questions in a letter, or uses a clinical advice form, will receive an appropriate and structured written response from the clinical advisor. This can then be passed directly to the lay chair, thus ensuring that both the convener and the lay chair have identical information available to them.

The medical records

As both the convener and the lay chair are lay people it is not necessary for them to have copies of the clinical records. It is the role of the clinical advisor to look at the clinical records to see if any additional information, which has not been passed onto the complainant, would help to address the outstanding issues.

An example would be when a complainant had complained about a delay in diagnosis and received the explanation that the practitioner was unable to confirm the diagnosis earlier and that the patient was given the diagnosis at the earliest possible time. The clinical advisor may state that the information given was correct but that it had omitted to give information on the number and type of tests given, all of which had negative results. They could recommend that a meeting should take place between the complainant and practitioner in order to explain which tests had been done and why it was not possible to make an earlier diagnosis.

Making the Convening Decision

Independently, the convener and the lay chair should consider each of the outstanding issues in turn. They should look through the correspondence, notes of meetings and the written clinical advice.

It is usual for the convener to telephone the lay chair. In simple complaints involving only one or two outstanding issues the decision can often be made at this stage. In more complex complaints it may be necessary for the convener and the lay chair to meet.

It is essential that the convener does not try to influence the lay chair; the usual approach would be for them to discuss each outstanding issue in turn. The convener first asks for the lay chair's decision and reasons for the decision. If the convener and lay chair are in agreement they would move on to the next issue. If there is disagreement a discussion would take place but ultimately the convener has the final decision.

A file note should then be made of the discussion and a record placed in the complaints file.

Options available at the Convening Decision

Four options are available to the convener and the lay chair at the convening stage:

1. Refer back for further Local Resolution
2. Refuse the request for an Independent Review Panel
3. Agree to hold an Independent Review Panel
4. Ask the Health Authority whether it is necessary to refer to the appropriate professional body, the NHS tribunal or the police.

It is possible to have a combination of the above options when dealing with each complaint. Following the decision the convener would write to the complainant, the parties complained against and the Health Authority chief executive advising them of the decision.

Refer back for further Local Resolution

This option would take place if it was felt that further action could be taken under Local Resolution or if it was a new complaint, in which case it would have to be referred back to Local Resolution. In this instance, the convener would write to all parties, informing them of the decision and making suggestions for further action. This could include, for example, meetings, lay conciliation or explanations about particular aspects of the complaint. The convener should take care when wording this response to make sure that they do not inadvertently make two decisions, for example:

I have decided to turn down your request for an Independent Review Panel as I have decided to refer your case back to Local Resolution.

A better form of wording would be:

I have discussed your request for an Independent Review Panel with an independent lay chair and we have decided to refer your case back for further Local Resolution.

The second example offers only one option.

The convener is also required to advise the complainant that, if the further suggestions for Local Resolution do not resolve the complaint, they have a right to re-request an Independent Review Panel and that this should be done within 28 days of the final letter of Local Resolution.

Refuse the request for an Independent Review Panel

If all the aims of the complaints procedure have been met or there is no further action that can be taken, the decision may be to refuse the request for an Independent Review Panel. An example of the latter could be if there was a complaint about manner and attitude and there were no other persons present at the time of the incident. If one of the parties states that the other was rude and the person who was accused denies being rude it would be very difficult to add any further information as it would be a case of one person's word against the other's. This decision would be especially correct if the correspondence contained a statement apologising for the fact that the manner and attitude of the member of staff was felt by the complainant to be unsatisfactory.

When refusing a request for an Independent Review Panel the convener should indicate where the outstanding issue had been answered, for example:

I note in the letter from Dr X to you, dated 30th January, that the reason for the 3-hour delay before the doctor was able to visit you was the high number of emergency calls that weekend because of the flu epidemic. I also note that Dr X did apologise for the delay. After consulting with the independent lay chair we have decided that the explanation given to you in that letter was full and complete and we do not believe that any further information could be forthcoming from an Independent Review Panel. We have therefore decided to refuse your request for an Independent Review Panel on that point.

As the convener has refused the request for the Independent Review Panel it is necessary to include details of the complainant's right to contact the Ombudsman and his name, address and telephone number should therefore be included in the letter.

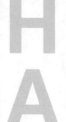
Health Authority

Agree to hold an Independent Review Panel

If the decision is to hold an Independent Review Panel then it is up to the convener to write the terms of reference for the panel. These should be based on those outstanding issues that require further explanation. In view of the fact that the Independent Review Panel is not a disciplinary panel, it is usual for the terms of reference to be open statements and time limited, for example:

To investigate Mrs X's care and treatment from 3 to 9 August.

To evaluate the out of hours visit to Mr Y on 10 September with particular reference to the administration arrangements for the call.

Although it is the convener's role to write the terms of reference, the responsibility for the Independent Review Panel rests with the independent lay chair. It is therefore good practice check the wording of the terms of reference with the lay chair before sending them out. The convener should then write to all parties advising them that a panel is being convened and enclosing the terms of reference for the panel.

Much discussion has taken place as to whether or not the terms of reference should be agreed with the complainant. Bearing in mind that they are based on the outstanding issues, as identified by the complainant, and that it is not possible to investigate any new issues at the Independent Review Panel stage, it seems reasonable that the final decision is the convener's. The trend appears to be that, once agreed with the lay chair, the terms of reference are sent to the complainant with a request to notify the convener if there are any comments.

Ask the Health Authority whether referral is necessary

If, at first sight, it appears that there are grounds for concern about the safety of patients, the convener should refer the case to the appropriate person in the Health Authority to decide whether to take action. If part, or all, of the complaint is referred to the appropriate professional body, the NHS tribunal or the police, then the complainant should be advised that no further action will be taken under the complaints procedure with regard to that aspect of the complaint. Any aspect of the complaint not referred for action is treated in the same way as a normal request for an Independent Review Panel.

If the Health Authority decides that no action will take place then the regulations state that 'a panel may be appointed'.

The convener should not look at cases to see if the Health Authority should initiate disciplinary action. The guidance states that the need for local disciplinary action should be considered only when the handling of a complaint has been concluded. Therefore action should be taken only if it is necessary to protect patients.

IF THE COMPLAINANT DISAGREES WITH THE CONVENER'S DECISION

The complainant does not have the right to have an Independent Review Panel. If the complainant does not wish to go back to Local Resolution, that is their right, but once the Convening Decision has been made it should not be changed. Therefore, if the complainant chooses not to go back to Local Resolution then the complaints procedure stops. Providing the convener's recommendations for further Local Resolution were reasonable then the complainant would usually be advised that the Ombudsman could not get involved as Local Resolution had not been completed.

If the complainant disagrees with the convener's decision to refuse a panel they have the right to go to the Ombudsman. If the Ombudsman felt that the correct process had not been followed he may invite the convener to reconsider the decision. This could happen if, for example, the convener had not taken clinical advice. The convener would then go through the decision-making process again, taking clinical advice. The final decision may or may not be the same.

CORRESPONDENCE AT THE CONVENING STAGE

The following correspondence is usually sent during the convening process.

- An initial acknowledgement letter from the complaints manager
- An appointment letter to the lay chair (as outlined on page 100)
- An acknowledgement letter to the complainant from the convener (sent within 2 days)
- A letter from the convener to the person complained against, informing them of the outstanding issues identified by the complainant
- A letter from the convener to the clinical advisor(s) outlining the process
- A letter from the convener to the lay chair outlining the process
- A file note of the discussion that takes place between the convener and the lay chair
- A letter from the convener to the complainant giving information concerning the final decision
- A letter from the convener to the parties complained against giving their final decision
- A letter to the chief executive.

Health Authority

Initial acknowledgement letter

It is recommended that receipt of the initial letter requesting an Independent Review Panel is acknowledged by the Health Authority. The acknowledgement letter would indicate that the request had been received and was being passed on to the convener, who would also acknowledge receipt of the request.

Acknowledgement letter from the convener to the complainant

This letter should be sent within 2 working days of the request being received by the convener. The following information may be included in the letter:

- An explanation on the position of the convener, stressing their impartiality
- A request to confirm the complainant's outstanding issues from Local Resolution (if this has not already been done)
- Information concerning consultation with the independent lay chair
- That the convener will be taking independent clinical advice
- The aims behind the Convening Decision
- That the convener cannot award compensation
- That if legal action is started the complaints procedure must stop
- That an Independent Review Panel cannot recommend disciplinary action
- That the options open to the convener are to: refer back to Local Resolution; refuse a panel; convene an Independent Review Panel
- That the time limit for the Convening Decision is 10 working days.

Letter from the convener to the person complained against

This letter advises the person complained against that a request for an Independent Review Panel has been received. The following information may be included in the letter:

- An explanation on the position of the convener, stressing their impartiality
- Information concerning consultation with the independent lay chair
- That the convener will be taking independent clinical advice
- The aims behind the Convening Decision
- That the convener cannot award compensation
- That if legal action is started the complaints procedure must stop

- That an Independent Review Panel cannot recommend disciplinary action
- That the options open to the convener are to: refer back to Local Resolution; refuse a panel; convene an Independent Review Panel
- That the time limit for the Convening Decision is 10 working days.

The letter could also include:

- A request for the practitioner to identify the section of the patient's records appropriate to the complaint
- An indication that the practitioner can get help and advice from the Local Representative Committee, the Medical Defence Union and the Medical Protection Society.

It is usual to enclose a copy of the complainant's letter stating the outstanding issues. The Health Service Circular *NHS Complaints Procedures: Confidentiality*, serial number HSC 1998/059, suggests that some conveners have circulated the complainant's statement to other parties and states that this should be done only in exceptional circumstances. It goes on to say that the statement should be sent to:

- the person who is subject to the complaint
- any other person named in the complaint
- the lay chair
- the clinical advisor(s).

If a panel is appointed the statement should also be sent to the panel members and the clinical assessors.

Letter from the convener to the clinical advisor

This letter is sent to each person who is acting as a clinical advisor to the convener. Some conveners ask their clinical advisors to complete a form so that the procedure is standardized. A copy of the form can then be passed on to the lay chair, ensuring that both parties responsible for the Convening Decision receive identical information.

The following information may be included in a letter requesting clinical advice:

- A copy of the outstanding issues from Local Resolution
- A request to concentrate on the outstanding areas, as outlined by the complainant
- A reminder that their comments are for the convener and the lay chair, both of whom are lay people, with a request that any medical terminology is explained
- A request to say whether or not the complainant has received a full explanation

Health Authority

- If the complainant has not received a full explanation and additional information is available, whether or not they have any further suggestions for Local Resolution
- Whether an apology is required and, if the answer is yes, has it been given?
- If an error has occurred, have satisfactory steps been put in place to prevent it happening again and has the complainant been fully advised about the action taken by the practice?
- A reminder that if an Independent Review Panel is refused the substance of the clinical advice will be passed on to the complainant.

Appended to the letter would be the correspondence and associate paper work from Local Resolution and the appropriate clinical records.

Letter from the convener to the lay chair

As conveners work in slightly different ways, it is helpful if the convener writes to the lay chair explaining how they work and what they expect of the lay chair. The following information may be included in such a letter:

- The name and contact details of the convener
- Whether Convening Decision forms are to be used
- A request for the lay chair to look at the outstanding issues and make a decision
- Information as to whether the decision could be made on the telephone or if a meeting is required
- The clinical advice received by the convener
- Details of who to contact if any further information is required
- An indication of who is to make the next contact and when.

File note

The file note usually contains the following information:

- The name of the lay chair and the convener
- The case reference
- The date the decision was made
- Whether it was a telephone conversation or a meeting
- The decision on each outstanding issue
- If there was agreement or disagreement about the outcome
- The date and signature of both parties.

This note would form part of the audit trail. It is a record of the Convening Decision and would be filed in the complaint's file.

Letter from the convener to the complainant giving the Convening Decision

The content of the letter would vary slightly depending on the result of the Convening Decision. It would usually inform the complainant:

- That consultation had taken place with an independent lay chair
- That clinical advice had been taken (if appropriate)
- Of the Convening Decision for each of the outstanding issues
- Of their rights following the Convening Decision.

If the complaint had been referred back to Local Resolution the letter would include:

- Suggestions for further action by the practice, for example lay conciliation
- A paragraph telling the complainant that they have the right to re-request an Independent Review Panel if further Local Resolution is unsuccessful.

If the request for an Independent Review Panel has been refused the letter would include:

- Information as to where the complaint had been answered
- The substance of the clinical advice
- A paragraph telling the complainant that they have the right to go to the Ombudsman and full information about how he can be contacted.

If the request for the Independent Review Panel had been agreed the letter would include the terms of reference for the panel.

Letter from the convener to the parties complained against

Following the Convening Decision the convener should write to all of the parties complained against:

- Advising them of the decision
- Outlining any further action required (if appropriate)
- Enclosing a copy of the letter to the complainant.

Letter to the chief executive

Following the Convening Decision the convener should write to the chief executive of the Health Authority:

- Advising them of the decision
- Outlining any further action required (if appropriate)
- Enclosing a copy of the letter to the complainant.

Health Authority

If the Convening Decision is to convene an Independent Review Panel, the letter should also advise the chief executive of:

• The terms of reference of the panel
• The need to appoint a third panel member
• Whether or not there is a need to appoint clinical assessors
• The need for administrative support for the panel.

13

The Independent Review Panel

An Independent Review Panel is made up of three members: the Health Authority's convener, the lay chair and a third lay member appointed by the Regional Office. If the complaint has a clinical component then the panel will be assisted by a minimum of two clinical assessors who are appointed from outside the Health Authority area.

PAPERWORK AND POLICIES

Prior to any Independent Review Panel a basic set of information will be required. Once obtained, this paperwork can be used for any subsequent panel that may be established. The paperwork will cover:

- Indemnity
- Confidentiality

- Expressions of interest
- Return and storage of papers
- Payable expenses
- Letters of appointment
- Secretarial support for the panel
- Tape-recording
- Panel papers, including medical records.

Indemnity

The lay chair, clinical assessors and purchaser representative will all require indemnity. This is provided by the Health Authority and should be signed by the chief executive. Typical wording in the appointment letter could be as follows:

A chairman or non-executive member or member who has acted honestly and in good faith will not have to meet out of his or her own personal resources any personal civil liability that is incurred in the execution or purported execution of his or her board function, save where the person has acted recklessly.

Confidentiality

Health Service Circular HSC 1999/053 *For the Record* discusses the management of records within Health Authorities. Section 4 of the circular emphasises the importance of maintaining professional ethical standards of confidentiality. The report discusses the confidential duty of people with access to patient information to the patient whose information they hold and goes on to stress that the duty of confidence is long established in common law.

The Caldicott Review of Patient Identifiable Information, published in December 1997, identified a general lack of awareness of confidentiality and information security throughout the NHS. Whereas the clinical assessors should be aware of the need for confidentiality through their professional training, the Health Authority will have a duty of care to ensure that the lay chair and the panel members do not disclose confidential information to unauthorised parties and that any paperwork is kept secure and safe at all times and is not accessible to any unauthorised person.

It will be up to each individual Health Authority to decide the amount of information given to ensure that confidentiality will be upheld. For example:

All activity undertaken under this appointment is confidential and should not be disclosed to any third parties. There may be circumstances when you are approached directly for information or comment about the panel's activities. All such approaches should be immediately referred to the Health Authority's ... manager.

Or:

Confidentiality:

1. The contents of the Independent Review Panel papers must not be discussed with anyone who is not directly involved in the Independent Review Panel process.
2. The papers should be kept in a safe and secure place and should be inaccessible to unauthorised persons at all times.
3. All papers should be returned to the Health Authority's ... manager on completion of the Independent Review Panel Report for safe storage.
4. The identity of the complainant must not be revealed to any person who is not directly involved in the Independent Review Panel process.

Expressions of interest

Before any papers are sent out to the panel members and the assessors, a check should be made to ensure that they do not know the parties involved in the complaint. This check can take the form of a telephone conversation. Problems may arise with clinical assessors, particularly if one of the staff involved in the complaint is well known in their field. The informal test has tended to be whether or not they would see the person socially, or invite them to their house.

The Health Authority therefore needs a method of working to make sure that these checks do take place and to clearly identify both the person doing the checks and the person sending out the papers. If this is not the same person then the responsibility for checking would usually rest with the person sending out the papers.

Return and storage of papers

As the Department of Health has indicated that complaints papers should be stored for the same length of time as medical records, a system needs to be in place outlining how and when the papers are returned and who is responsible for checking that this has been done.

Some lay chairs have argued that they wish to keep their papers in case the complaint is referred to the Health Services Commissioner. Perhaps the simplest way of handling this is to suggest that they place their personal notes in a sealed envelope and put their name and the complaint reference on the outside. This can then be filed with the complaints papers and returned if required. Any duplicate papers should be destroyed by Health Authority staff. It is not acceptable to allow the panel members or assessors to destroy their own papers as the Health Authority will have no means of knowing that this has been done correctly.

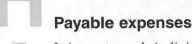

Payable expenses

It is up to each individual Health Authority to decide the rate at which expenses are reimbursed. Guidance was issued by the Head of Employment Issues at the NHS Executive Headquarters in September 1996 and the payment to panel members and clinical assessors was covered in EL(96)19. Panel chairs are eligible for travel expenses, subsistence allowance and loss of earnings. Conveners who are non-executive directors cannot receive any additional payment but it is up to Health Authorities to make their own arrangement when appointing additional conveners.

Clinical assessors can claim an honorarium of £150 per day (consultant medical and dental staff can claim £175), along with travel and subsistence allowance.

It is helpful to the panel members and assessors if, on appointment, information is sent from the Health Authority outlining:

- The rate at which travel allowance is paid
- Whether additional expenditures can be claimed (e.g. telephone, postage)
- What is acceptable as loss of earnings and what documentation will be required, possibly with a maximum daily rate payable
- The payment rate for clinical assessors
- Whether overnight accommodation will be provided.

In addition, a travel and subsistence claim form should be provided, with details of when and to whom it should be returned.

Letters of appointment

These can take the form of a standard letter and should be sent out immediately after the appointments have been agreed and it has been confirmed that the parties do not have an interest in the case. The letter would contain some or all of the following information.

- The name of the complainant
- The subject of the complaint
- Confirmation of the appointment
- An indication that the Independent Review Panel is a subcommittee of the Health Authority
- Indemnity information
- Confidentiality information
- Reimbursement of travel, subsistence, postage, fee (for clinical assessors), amount paid for loss of earnings (lay chairs, if appropriate)
- A request to confirm that they do not have an interest
- A statement that they agree to the conditions outlined in the letter

- A request to date and sign one copy and return it to the Health Authority, retaining the other copy for their records
- A copy of the *Briefing Pack for Clinical Assessors* produced by the Institute of Health and Care Development and published by the NHS Executive (for clinical assessors).

Secretarial support for the panel

If the Health Authority's complaints manager has been dealing with the complaint under Local Resolution it is advisable for another person to provide the secretarial and administrative support for the panel. This distances the Independent Review Panel from the Local Resolution process. In some larger Health Authorities, with more than one complaints manager, one will deal with Local Resolution and the other with the Independent Review Panel. In smaller Health Authorities, someone who can support the panel needs to be identified at the beginning of the process. This person will need to have the time to administer all correspondence and to take minutes at any panel meetings, bearing in mind the time scales laid down for the completion of each stage of the process.

All meetings of the panel should be minuted so that an audit trail can take place. If the complaint is subsequently referred to the Ombudsman, these minutes will be required if the complaint is investigated.

Tape-recording

Whether or not the Independent Review Panel's work should be tape-recorded is a decision for each individual Health Authority. Before a decision is taken, the following points should be considered:

- Why is recording necessary?
- Will the tape be transcribed?
- If yes, will the transcriber be able to recognise who is speaking?
- If no, is the recording a back-up to the minute taker?
- Will the parties be informed in advance about the recording?
- What will happen if someone refuses to be recorded?
- What will happen if the machine jams?
- What will happen to the tape after the Independent Review Panel?
- What is the Health Authority's position if they are asked for a copy of the tape?

If the decision is made to tape-record proceedings it is advisable to inform the parties well in advance that this will be happening. The Health Authority should ask their permission and advise them of the purpose of the tape-recording and what will happen to the tape at the end of the Independent Review Panel process.

Health Authority

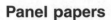

Health Authority

Panel papers

The panel members and the clinical assessors will require the following papers prior to the Independent Review Panel.

• The terms of reference
• Copies of any correspondence concerning the complaint
• Notes of any Local Resolution meetings
• Patient records relevant to the complaint
• Nursing records relevant to the complaint (if appropriate).

The correspondence and notes of any meetings should be numbered and in date order as this aids discussion at any subsequent meetings. A cover sheet listing the correspondence is useful as it makes it much easier to find a particular piece of correspondence when required.

The papers need to be sent out as soon as possible after the request for an Independent Review Panel has been granted. Included with the papers should be:

• Dates and times of any subsequent meetings
• Details of the venue
• A map of the venue
• Information concerning contact names and telephone numbers.

Care should be taken to ensure that the papers arrive safely. Boxes or Jiffy bags are preferable to standard envelopes, as the latter often become damaged in transit.

It is advisable to mark the packaging in such a way as to indicate that the contents are confidential and that the package should be opened only by the addressee.

THE LAY CHAIR

Once the Convening Decision has been made to convene an Independent Review Panel, and the terms of reference have been written, the responsibility moves from the convener to the lay chair. The Health Authority is required to provide administrative support for the lay chair. The role of the lay chair is to:

• Chair any meetings of the panel
• Decide, in conjunction with the panel members, how the panel should operate
• Resolve any disagreement about the procedure to be adopted
• Question those interviewed, as appropriate
• Lead the panel in writing its report
• Ensure that there are no suggestions or recommendations about disciplinary action in the report
• Agree the draft circulation of the report with the panel members

- Aim to meet the target time scales for the Independent Review Panel
- Decide if, in the interest of the patient, part of the report should be withheld
- Sign and distribute the final report.

THE LAY PANEL MEMBER

The role of the lay panel member is to:

- Read the papers
- Participate in any meetings of the panel
- Decide, with the lay chair, how the panel should do its work
- Question those interviewed, as appropriate
- Contribute to the report of the panel
- Agree, with the lay chair, the distribution of the draft report
- Check the final panel report.

THE CONVENER

The role of the convener is similar to that of the lay member, i.e. to:

- Read the papers
- Participate in any meetings of the panel
- Decide, with the lay chair, how the panel should do its work
- Question those interviewed, as appropriate
- Contribute to the panel's final report
- Agree, with the lay chair, the distribution of the draft report
- Check the final panel report.

CLINICAL ASSESSORS

The clinical assessors are appointed from outside the Health Authority area. In clinical complaints there must be at least two clinical assessors. They are selected from the list provided by the Regional Office and are appointed by the Local Representative Committee. If a complaint concerns only one profession then two assessors from that profession would be appointed. If the complaint concerns more than one profession then an assessor from each speciality would be required, for example a general practitioner and a nurse.

The role of the clinical assessors is to:

- Advise the panel on the clinical aspects of the terms of reference
- Produce draft reports prior to the panel hearing
- Participate in any meetings of the panel
- Question those interviewed, as appropriate

Health Authority

- Contribute to the report of the panel
- Check the final panel report
- Produce either an individual or joint clinical assessor's report using lay terminology.

A suggested content of the final assessor's report would be:

- A summary of the clinical aspects of the case
- The findings and recommendations for each of the terms of reference.

The clinical assessors *cannot* suggest disciplinary action.

SUGGESTED PROCEDURE FOR THE INDEPENDENT REVIEW PANEL PROCESS

There is no laid-down procedure for the Independent Review Panel process. This allows flexibility and enables the panel to accommodate the needs of individual complainants. Unfortunately, problems have arisen from this flexibility, as certain criteria must be upheld, for example:

- The complainant and the complained against must be treated equally
- Clinical assessors must be present when clinical issues are discussed
- The participants have to be allowed to put their case orally or, if they wish, in writing
- Any complainant can be accompanied by a relative or friend plus an advisor when interviewed
- Any person complained against can be accompanied by an advisor when interviewed
- Any interview has to be in private
- Notes should be kept of all interviews.

Therefore, although there is flexibility in the system, the majority of panels adopt the following procedure:

- A meeting of panel members as soon as it is known that a panel is to be convened
- An initial meeting of the panel and clinical assessors immediately prior to the Independent Review Panel
- The Independent Review Panel
- A meeting immediately after the Independent Review Panel.

A meeting of panel members as soon as it is known that a panel is to be convened

This meeting involves the panel members only and gives them an opportunity to meet each other. As with all meetings of the panel, a record should be kept of the panel's discussions. At this meeting the following information can be decided:

- Which practitioners and staff will need to be interviewed
- Whether written statements can be taken
- Whether any additional papers are required
- The order in which the interviews will take place
- The length of time allocated to each interview
- The venue for the Independent Review Panel
- The date for the Independent Review Panel
- If there are any exceptional circumstances that need to be taken into account.

Experience shows that it usually takes between 1 and 2 hours for the complainant to give information to the panel and between 15 minutes and 1 hour for practitioners and staff. The length of time required will depend on the complexity of the case.

Who can attend?

A relative or friend plus a person to act as an advisor can accompany the complainant. If more than one family member is involved in the complaint then they all attend the Independent Review Panel together. The person accompanying may speak to the panel with the lay chair's consent but, if they are legally qualified, they may not act as an advocate. It should be remembered that the aim of the panel is to establish what happened and therefore first-hand accounts will always carry more weight than second-hand accounts.

The practitioner may also be accompanied by an advisor, who could be a member of the Local Representative Committee, the Medical Defence Union or the Medical Protection Society. It is usual to see the practitioners and staff individually.

It is usual for the complainant to be interviewed first and then the practitioner. This is much less confrontational than having both parties in together and appears to allow a much more open dialogue between the panel and the person being interviewed. It has been argued that the complainant may wish to hear what the practitioner and staff are saying to the panel but there are facilities for this to happen under Local Resolution and they will have a summary of the information given to the panel in the final report.

Accommodation required for the panel

The venue for the Independent Review Panel is often at the Health Authority. Ideally, the room should be large enough to seat the panel

Health Authority

Health Authority

members, clinical assessors, secretarial support, the complainant and their relatives, friends and advisor.

It is much easier if everyone can sit round the same table. This allows people to place any papers on the table and allows the panel members and the parties being interviewed to take notes if they wish. It has been argued that the use of low chairs and coffee tables is a better arrangement but this can give an appearance of informality and the impression that the panel is not taking the complaint seriously.

The provision of separate waiting areas where the parties can speak to their advisors prior to coming into the review is often appreciated, as is the provision of beverages and name plates for the panel members and assessors.

The list provided in Chapter 3 (p. 18) with suggestions for access for disabled people could be used to check the suitability of the chosen venue; the information on the use of interpreters (also in Chapter 3; p. 17) should also be noted.

Exceptional circumstances

There may be occasions when it is not appropriate for the complainant to appear before the full panel. An example would be if the patient was bedridden, very elderly or had learning difficulties and it was thought that a panel would be intimidating. In these circumstances it would be possible for one of the panel members to interview the complainant on their own. If the complaint had a clinical nature they would have to be accompanied by one of the clinical assessors. Minutes of the meeting would be recorded and the information fed back to the other panel members.

If the panel was arranged and, on the day, one of the panel members was unable to attend due to illness or an unavoidable situation, it is still possible for the panel to go ahead, rather than cancelling and reconvening the meeting. If the lay chair was unable to attend it would be more acceptable for the lay member to chair the panel than the convener, as they would be seen to be more independent. If one of the clinical assessors was unable to attend, the panel could still go ahead but this should be the exception rather than normal procedure.

Performance targets

Performance targets are laid down in the Guidance documentation and are as follows:

- Appointment of panel members – 10 working days after the Convening Decision
- Draft report of the panel – 30 working days after the panel has been set up

- Final panel report – a further 10 working days
- Report sent to the complainant by the Health Authority chief executive – a further 20 working days.

The performance targets are for guidance only. If they are not going to be met then all the parties should be informed that there will be a delay and given the reasons for the delay. It is the lay chair's responsibility to maintain time scales, although, in reality, the monitoring is usually done by Health Authority staff.

An initial meeting of the panel and clinical assessors immediately prior to the Independent Review Panel

This meeting usually takes place for about an hour immediately prior to the Independent Review Panel. Each clinical assessor usually produces a draft report based on the written documentation and clinical records. At this meeting the draft assessor's reports are discussed and the order of questioning is agreed. It is usual for the clinical assessors to concentrate on the clinical aspect of the complaint and at this meeting will decide if they will answer questions posed to them by the complainant and if they will explain certain areas of the case to the complainant. Both the answering of questions and the provision of explanations will often help the complainant understand what has happened. The fact that the explanation comes from someone outside the practice is often more acceptable than the same explanation given by the practice staff. In addition, as the interview is minuted there will be a record of the answers and explanations, which will allow the complainant to re-read the information at a later date.

It is usual for the lay chair to sit in the centre of the panel with a panel member and clinical assessor on either side.

The Independent Review Panel

As has already been mentioned, the running of the panel is not laid down but the most common approach is to interview the complainant first, followed by the complained against and any other members of the staff the panel require to see. By far the most usual procedure is as follows:

- The lay chair meets the person to be interviewed outside the room
- The lay chair brings the person into the room and introduces them to the panel members and the assessors
- The lay chair explains the procedure
- The lay chair reads out the terms of reference for the panel
- The lay chair invites the person being interviewed to outline any information they wish to tell the panel

Health Authority

- The clinical assessors ask questions
- The panel members ask questions
- The lay chair explains the next stage in the procedure and thanks the person for attending.

Greeting the interviewee

Usually, the lay chair goes to meet the person being interviewed. This gives them a brief opportunity to meet all the people involved. Introductions can be made and the lay chair can indicate that they are independent from the Health Authority. The lay chair then brings the participants into the room and introduces the panel members and clinical assessors, indicating who they are, where they are from and their role on the panel.

The procedure

After sitting down, the lay chair explains how the panel will operate, indicating that the panel wishes to hear the individual's account of what happened and that then they will be interviewing the staff involved. The person minuting the panel is introduced and the interviewee is informed that they will have an opportunity to see the minutes of the information they give to the panel for approval before the report is published.

The terms of reference

Reading out the terms of reference reminds the person being interviewed and the panel members of the parameters of the panel. This hopefully allows the panel to concentrate on the areas of importance and prevents extra issues, or those that have been answered under Local Resolution, being introduced at this stage of the proceedings.

The opening statement

Asking the interviewee to give their account of what happened allows them to tell their story. It is helpful if they can be allowed to speak without interruption as this enables them to feel that they have had the opportunity to say what they want to say. Many people see the Independent Review Panel as their 'day in court' and have often rehearsed what they want to say. In cases of bereavement this can often be a very emotional time for them and the provision of water and paper tissues can help. In some cases the telling of the story is a form of release and can sometimes help a bereaved person through that stage of the bereavement process.

Health Authority

The questions

Once the interviewee has made their statement, the panel members and clinical assessors have an opportunity to ask them questions. The panel members should bear in mind that part of the panel report is the findings of fact about the terms of reference. Therefore closed questions are often a useful way of clarifying the facts of the complaint. For example:

- Did the Doctor examine you?
- Did you ask to speak to the Doctor?
- Which nurse did you speak to?
- Which day did you visit?
- What time did you telephone?

This is also an opportunity for the clinical assessors to answer questions from the interviewee and to explain areas of concern that the interviewee may have.

The closing remarks

The lay chair thanks the interviewees for attending and explains the next stages. This may include.

- Giving information on the time scales
- Telling them that they will see the minutes of the interview
- Reminding them that the report is confidential
- Informing them of their right to go to the Ombudsman
- Offering condolences if a bereavement has occurred.

The whole procedure is then repeated for each person being interviewed.

A meeting immediately after the Independent Review Panel

Although in complex complaints the panel can be very tired by this point in the proceedings, it is very useful and effective to have a meeting with the panel members and the clinical assessors to discuss:

- The findings of fact
- The opinions of the panel
- Recommendations.

The findings of fact

The findings of fact are numbered and written in date order. They provide a summary of the case pertaining to the terms of reference. Events can be listed as fact when both parties agree or when they are supported by

Health Authority

contemporaneous written evidence or by an independent person. Practitioners are used to summarising information and can be invaluable in this stage of the process. For example:

1. On 10 September Mr Smith returned home from hospital after undergoing radiotherapy for carcinoma of the pharynx.

2. When Mr Smith arrived home he vomited and felt ill, his wife telephoned the surgery at 2 p.m. and requested a visit. She was told to ring back in an hour as the doctor was visiting patients.

3. Mrs Smith rang back at 3 p.m. and was asked to ring back again in an hour as the doctor had not returned.

4. Mrs Smith rang at 4 p.m. and was told that the doctor would visit after evening surgery.

5. The doctor arrived at 6.15 p.m., he did not examine the patient and no record of the consultation was made at the time. He advised Mr Smith to take small sips of water and to attend for radiotherapy the following day.

The opinions of the panel

The panel members and the assessors then take each term of reference in turn and discuss it, based on the findings of fact. For example:

• To evaluate the out-of-hours visit to Mr Smith on 10 September with particular reference to the administration arrangements for the call.

The panel were advised by the clinical assessors that there was no record of the visit made by the doctor in the patient's records. They expressed concern about the number of telephone calls that Mrs Smith had to make and the lack of treatment offered. The panel were concerned that there did not appear to be a system for contacting the practitioner when they were away from the practice or visiting patients.

The recommendations

When making recommendations the panel has to remember that the Independent Review Panel is a subcommittee of the Health Authority and that they should not suggest any disciplinary action. Recommendations should therefore suggest ways in which the practice could improve the services it offers, or improve the efficiency or effectiveness of the practice. In addition, the panel could make recommendations as to ways in which the practice could satisfy the complainant. For example, the panel could recommend that:

1. The practitioner considers the use of a mobile telephone or paging system so that contact could be maintained with the practice during on-call visits.

2. The practitioner ensures that a contemporaneous record is kept of all patient visits.

THE CLINICAL ASSESSOR REPORTS

The clinical assessors can produce individual reports or a joint report. Some Health Authorities offer facilities for the assessors to dictate their final reports on the day but this will depend on the complexity of the Independent Review Panel. Separate reports are seen as being more independent by the complainant but care should be taken to make sure that any contradictory sections are clearly explained and to indicate why there is a difference of opinion.

Joint reports can run the risk of the clinicians being accused of colluding but can be helpful in very complex complaints to help clarify, in a logical manner, the clinical aspects of the case.

THE INDEPENDENT REVIEW PANEL REPORT

The final, confidential report is produced by the panel. There are certain compulsory elements to the report, which are outlined in the underpinning legislation and include:

- The findings of fact relevant to the complaint
- The opinion of the panel on the findings of fact
- The reasons for the panel's opinion
- The assessor's report
- If the panel disagrees with any aspect of the assessor's report, the reason for the disagreement.

Comments from the Ombudsman in his annual reports have indicated further information to be included in the final report. In addition, summaries of papers received by the panel members and a summary of evidence given to the panel makes the report into a document that can be read and understood as a document in its own right. The suggested format of the report is shown in Figure 13.1.

The draft report

There has been much discussion as to whether a draft report should be sent to the parties involved. It is argued that issuing a draft report gives people the opportunity to correct any errors before the final report is published. The problems associated with the issuing of a full draft report are related to how the panel deals with any corrections:

- What would the panel do if the complainant wished to change someone else's statement?

Health Authority

CONFIDENTIAL

Name of Health Authority/HA
Report of the Independent Review Panel
held on (date)

Complaint brought by............

Panel Members
> Name   Position

Clinical Assessors
> Name   Position

Terms of Reference
> List

Panel Procedure
> A brief summary of the steps the panel took to investigate the complaint, including any meetings held and a list of documentation reviewed by the panel.

Précis of Interviews/Written Statements
> Covering only the information relevant to the terms of reference.

*Findings of Fact
> Numbered and in date order.

*Opinions of the panel on the Findings of Fact
> Take each of the terms of reference and comment, based on the findings of fact and giving reasons for any observations. If a finding of fact cannot be found, give the reasons.

If the panel disagrees with any matter included in the assessor's report
> Give reasons for the disagreements.

Recommendations
> The panel recommends to the Health Authority (if appropriate).

Signature
> Of lay chair (and other panel members if desired).

Date

Appendices

* Clinical Assessor's Report(s)
> Signed and dated

> *** Mandatory as per the directions**

Fig. 13.1

- How would the panel react if they disagreed with the 'correction'?
- What would the panel do if one person wanted a finding of fact changed but another agreed with the original version?

It could be argued that if the panel is not going to act on the changes identified then it is not appropriate to send out the full draft report. In addition, there is the potential for having two reports in circulation – the draft report and the final report. It would therefore be sensible to mark the draft report very clearly, so there can be no confusion at a later date.

A compromise has been found to work very well. The person who was interviewed receives a copy of the full minutes of their interview for checking. Any corrections are accepted by the panel. The corrected report is then summarised to exclude any new areas that are outside the terms of reference and the summarised version is included in the final report.

ISSUES ARISING DURING THE INDEPENDENT REVIEW PANEL PROCESS

As has been stated earlier, the purpose of the complaints process is to provide a full explanation to the complainant; it is not to lay blame or to suggest disciplinary action – the panel and assessors must remain impartial and both parties should be treated equally and fairly. It has to be remembered that in order to be granted an Independent Review Panel the complainant must state what issues remain outstanding and why they remain dissatisfied; the terms of reference for the Independent Review Panel arise from these outstanding issues. Therefore, originally it is the complainant who determines which issues form the basis of the panel's deliberations.

Several problem areas have arisen during and after Independent Review Panels:

- The introduction of new issues by the complainant
- The introduction of areas of concern by the clinical assessors
- The naming of people in the body of the report.

The introduction of new areas by the complainant

The directions are very clear and state that any new issues should be referred back to Local Resolution. However, once the panel procedure is under way this is very difficult to do. A practical way of handling this is for the lay chair to allow any queries to be answered, usually by one of the clinical assessors. As this discussion will be minuted, and the complainant will see the full minutes they will therefore have a written copy of the explanation given. However, the account included in the final report would cover only the areas included in the terms of reference for the panel, and not this new area.

The introduction of areas of concern by the clinical assessors

One of the problems in handling complaints is that the complainant some-times complains about the wrong person or the wrong area. As the purpose of the panel is to answer the complaint, how should any areas of concern be handled? The answer will depend on the severity of the areas under concern. It should be remembered that it is very easy to find areas for improvement when reviewing someone else's work as it is impossible for anyone to provide a 'gold standard' service 100% of the time. It will be for the clinical assessors to advise the panel if their concerns are such that further action needs to be taken, bearing in mind that they have a duty of care to report any serious areas of concern. What must be remembered is that if the areas of concern are outside the terms of reference for the panel then the panel report is not the place to raise these concerns. They should therefore be raised with either the chief executive or the medical director of the Health Authority concerned.

The naming of people in the body of the report

The question then arises as to whether or not the parties should be named in the body of the report. The *Guidance on Implementing the NHS Complaints Procedure* advises that when anonymised information would suffice, any identifiable information should be omitted. The Ombudsman names the complainant and the Health Authority in his reports but does not name the individuals interviewed, referring to them only by their job title. It has been argued, usually by lay chairs, that the parties should be named, as the process should be open and transparent.

Before naming individuals in a report the following questions should be asked:

- Is it fair for a member of staff to be named if they are correctly following a practice policy but that the policy or procedure is incorrect?
- Does it add to the provision of a full explanation to the patient if the staff are named?
- Will it improve the service to other patients if staff are named?
- Would the staff be being treated equitably if they are named in the report?

H A

Health Authority

- What would the Health Authority's position be if the staff are named and the report is published in the press?

CIRCULATION OF THE FINAL REPORT

Copies of the final report are sent to:
The chief executive of the Health Authority, who in turn sends them out to:

- The complainant
- Any person complained against
- Any person interviewed
- The patient, if they are not the complainant
- The assessors
- The chair of the Health Authority.

It is possible for the lay chair to withold parts of the report in the interest of protecting the confidentiality of the patient and any third party, or of protecting the health of the complainant or a patient who is not the complainant.

Any written statements provided to the panel should not be disclosed unless the person providing the information has consented to the disclosure and the Guidance clearly states that when anonymised information about patients or third parties would suffice then identifiable information should be omitted.

HSC 1998/059, issued to lay chairs, indicates that the full report should be seen by a limited number of people. It quotes the example that if the panel interviews people who are not directly involved in the complaint, then they should only see the parts of the report that relate to the information they gave, and not the full report. If the lay chair decides to withhold part of the report then it would be sensible to record the reasons for that decision.

THE COVERING LETTER

The final report has to be sent out by the chief executive within 5 working days of its receipt. A covering letter should explain that both parties have a right to complain to the Ombudsman and provide contact details. If the panel has made recommendations then the chief executive should invite the practitioner to write to the complainant advising them of the action taken by the practice. In addition, the chief executive should write to the complainant advising them of this request. It is helpful if the letter can indicate that the report is confidential. Once the report has been circulated, the lay chair should have no further contact with the parties involved.

Health Authority

ACTION FOLLOWING THE DISSEMINATION OF THE FINAL REPORT

If the chief executive considers that the content of the report indicates that disciplinary action may be required, a Health Authority reference panel will be set up. This panel is made up of at least one non-executive and one executive member of the Authority, plus one other person and a clinical advisor. The reference committee decides whether any further action is required, for example retraining, or if a disciplinary panel is required.

If it is decided to take disciplinary action the Health Authority becomes the complainant and the case is heard by a neighbouring Health Authority. Information gathered during Local Resolution belongs to the practice and therefore cannot be accessed by the Health Authority. The Guidance indicates that information obtained during the Independent Review Process cannot routinely be used in disciplinary investigations.

14

Complaints monitoring and Clinical Governance

STATISTICAL REPORTS

The Health Authority should collect statistics on the number of:

- Complaints dealt with by each practice
- Purchasing complaints received
- Cases dealt with by the conciliator(s)
- Independent Review Panel requests received
- Independent Review Panels held.

The Trusts within the Health Authority's boundaries should produce an annual report on complaints handling and copies of these reports should be sent to the Health Authority. These reports may include details of the:

- Number of complaints received
- Time taken to handle the complaints
- Number of Independent Review Panel requests received
- Time taken for the Convening Decision
- Number of Independent Review Panels held.

These reports are required to enable Health Authorities to:

- Monitor complaint handling
- Identify trends in complaints
- Identify areas for service improvements
- Consider lessons that can be learnt from complaints.

STATISTICS IN PRIMARY CARE

Health Authorities should know the name of the complaints manager for each primary care practice, the address where they can be contacted and information on how the practice complaints system is handled. Primary care practices do not have to supply detailed information about specific complaints and need only supply the Health Authority with the number of complaints that have been handled.

Conciliators are required to keep information about complaints confidential. They are, however, required to supply the Health Authority with information on the number of complaints they have handled and the results of the conciliation. These reports should be written in such a way as to ensure that neither the complainant nor the practice concerned can be identified.

THE INTERFACE BETWEEN COMPLAINTS AND CLINICAL GOVERNANCE

Purchasing complaints

Purchasing complaints should be monitored to identify trends and areas for concern. The frequency of monitoring will depend on the number of complaints received but it is advisable that it takes place at least every 6 months. To be objective, monitoring should involve people who are not directly involved in the complaints process or in handling this type of complaint. The use of a non-executive director and possible a CHC representative could bring an outside view to the process.

If systems require changing, the most effective way for this to be handled is for an action plan to be produced. This should clearly identify:

- What action is required
- Who is responsible for implementing the action
- When the work should be completed
- Who should monitor the progress
- How the final information is to be disseminated, and to whom.

Primary care complaints

As the Health Authority receives data concerning only the number of complaints received by a practice, it is not possible to use this route to effectively monitor performance. The number of complaints received may bear no relationship to the quality of care received by patients. If a practice is open, clearly advertises the complaints system and actually encourages comments, the number of complaints received may be high. These high numbers reflect an opportunity to improve services rather than a criticism of services. Alternatively, practices that do not advertise their complaints system, automatically remove patients who make a complaint and respond in a very negative way to complaints may well record very few complaints. In this instance, the patients may be getting a very poor service.

There may be occasions when external clinicians become involved in a complaint, either through their role as clinical advisors to the conciliator or through providing clinical advice to the convener. The issue to be addressed is, what action should be taken if they suspect poor clinical practice or they identify areas of poor practice that the complainant has not complained about? These potential areas of concern should be discussed with the Local Representative Committee and the Primary Care Group/Primary Care Trust/Health Authority before they arise and a protocol for handling such situations should be agreed. The practitioner should then be clear about the course of action to be taken if and when a situation arises.

Examples of such situations could include:

- Very poor but adequate record keeping
- Not acting on test results.

The course of action is determined by the part of the complaints procedure in which the situation arose. If an independent practitioner went to see a complainant with a conciliator and felt that, although information was recorded about each consultation, the information was barely adequate, it may be acceptable for the independent practitioner to discuss the record keeping (in private) with the practitioner, suggest ways in which it could be improved and give reasons why it was felt to be inadequate. How and where the contents of this conversation are recorded would be covered in the protocol. Either the independent practitioner could keep personal notes or a record could be passed to the appropriate clinical governance lead, the Primary Care Trust/Group, the Local Representative Committee chair or the Health Authority.

The course of action in the second example, where test results had not been acted upon, would depend on the severity of the incident. If the independent practitioner thought that other patients may be at risk then it may be necessary to invoke the mechanism for reporting the practitioner to the appropriate professional body. Alternatively, there may be a panel procedure where several people could look at the issues raised and instigate action that could include visiting the practitioner concerned. If the original concerns are substantiated then resultant action could include retraining, mentoring, professional support and advice or a full audit of practice procedure.

LEARNING FROM COMPLAINTS

Ideally, if people are to learn from complaints then the learning process should be wider than the individuals concerned. Perhaps the advent of Primary Care Groups and Trusts with their clinical governance leads could encourage practitioners to discuss complaints openly, to share the lessons learnt and to disseminate good practice. Anonymised articles or a regular column in a newsletter can be used for these purposes and could help to improve services and, in turn, reduce the number of complaints.

Complaints about purchasing

Although the method of handling complaints about purchasing is similar to that of handling Trust complaints, there are several areas of difference. This chapter will attempt to identify these.

WHO MAY COMPLAIN?

Anyone can complain about a Health Authority's purchasing decision but only those complaints that directly affect an individual patient come under the NHS complaints procedure. If complaints are received, for example from the general public, pressure groups or the CHC, these people are entitled to receive a full explanation about the decision-making process and the reasons why a particular decision was made. However, as this is not under the complaints procedure, they would not be entitled, for example, to request an Independent Review Panel.

Individual patients who have been affected by a purchasing decision may complain under the complaints procedure. The areas covered by these complaints usually centre round the rationing of drugs or services, for example, if a patient is refused infertility treatment because they do not meet the Health Authority's criteria or they have been told that they cannot have a particular drug as it is considered by the Health Authority to be not clinically effective.

LOCAL RESOLUTION

The complaint should be acknowledged by the complaints manager within two working days. The complaint should be investigated and a full response sent to the complainant within 20 working days; the response should be signed by the chief executive. It could suggest a meeting or lay conciliation if this was felt to be appropriate and that it would assist the complainant. Any meeting should be followed by a final letter from the chief executive summarising the information discussed at the meeting and answering any new questions that have been raised by the complainant. The final letter following Local Resolution should advise the complainant of their right to request an Independent Review Panel.

THE CONVENING DECISION

A request for an Independent Review Panel goes to the Health Authority's convener. Care must be taken to ensure that the convener does not have a conflict of interest in the case. If the convener is a non-executive director of the Health Authority they may well have approved, at a board meeting, the policy that is now being complained about. Consideration should therefore be given to appointing associate conveners to look at purchasing complaints or, alternatively, using a convener from a neighbouring Health Authority as an associate convener.

The convener would consult with a lay chair in the usual way and, if there is a clinical element to the complaint, they will need to take independent clinical advice. Again, as with the convener, the clinicians in the Public Health department may well have been involved in formulating the original policy and therefore the Regional Office will need to be contacted to provide the name of a clinical advisor.

THE INDEPENDENT REVIEW PANEL

It should be remembered that although panels may comment on the way the purchasing policy was formulated, if the correct criteria were used in writing the policy the panel will not be able to change the original policy. If, on the other hand, those formulating the policy had not consulted fully, if the policy was made on cost rather than clinical grounds or if there was insufficient clinical evidence to support the decision, the panel may well be able to comment.

The panel would comprise of the lay chair, the convener and a third panel member allocated by the Regional Office. If there is a clinical component to the complaint then the Regional Office will nominate two clinical assessors.

THE CIRCULATION OF THE FINAL REPORT

The lay chair sends out the final report. It is helpful if the letter can indicate that the report is confidential. Once the report has been circulated, the lay chair should have no further contact with the parties involved. Copies of the final report are sent to:

- The complainant
- Any person complained against
- Any person interviewed
- The patient, if they are not the complainant
- The assessors
- The chair and chief executive of the purchasing Health Authority
- The Regional Office of the NHS Executive.

ACTION FOLLOWING THE DISSEMINATION OF THE FINAL REPORT

Within 20 working days of the receipt of the report, the Health Authority chief executive should write to the complainant saying what action the Health Authority proposes to take following the panel's recommendations. If the Health Authority decides not to take any action on the recommendations then the reasons for this decision must be given. In addition, the complainant should be informed that they have the right to contact the Ombudsman if they remain dissatisfied; full contact details should be included in the letter.

TIME SCALES
Local Resolution

- Acknowledgement letter – 2 days
- Full response – 20 days
- Complainant to apply for Independent Review Panel – 28 days.

Independent Review

- Acknowledgement by the convener – 2 days
- Convening decision – 20 days
- Appointment of panel members – 20 days
- Draft panel report – 50 days
- Final panel report – 10 days
- Response to complainant – 20 days.

Health Authority

Secondary care complaints

16

Can complaints be prevented?

ANALYSIS OF INDEPENDENT REVIEW PANELS

When looking at Trust Independent Review Panel reports it was noted that 12 out of 21 involved the death of a patient. This finding implies that the way patients and relatives are handled before and after a bereavement is crucial. Further analysis indicated the following themes:

- Poor communication
- Poor record keeping
- Missed or late diagnosis
- Poor complaint handling.

Conveying bad news

It is never easy to tell a person that a relative has died or that they are suffering from a life-threatening illness. When undertaking this task the following guidance points may be of help:

The room

- The news should be given in private without interruptions from outside the room
- Tissues should be available
- Consider removing a white coat, especially if it is blood stained
- Tea- and coffee-making facilities and cold drinks should be available
- A mirror and wash basin in the room allows people to freshen up if they have been upset
- A telephone is useful to enable people to contact relatives, friends or neighbours without having to use a public telephone
- Unplug the telephone during the interview to avoid interruptions.

secondary care

2

Giving the news

- If the interview is to tell a patient bad news, ask them to bring a trusted friend or relative with them
- Check what the patient or relatives already know before giving further information
- Give the relative time to ask questions
- Remember that most patients do want to be told what is wrong with them
- Remember that a warning shot can be helpful (for example, I am afraid I have some bad news for you)
- Refer to a person who has died by name
- Watch and wait after breaking the news
- If the person becomes angry, remember that it may be a displacement for other forms of distress and therefore the anger should be acknowledged and not met with anger
- Do not leave relatives alone unless they request to be left alone. If so, tell them how to contact a member of staff
- Do not be ashamed to show your feelings – people often appreciate knowing that the doctor or nurse cared
- It may be appropriate to leave the relative with a nurse and then return in 30 minutes to answer questions
- The patient may cut short any explanation (e.g. I will leave all that to you, I will concentrate on getting better). If this happens, make a note in the records and return to the subject at the next consultation
- Consider giving only the most basic information when the relatives are first told, follow-up with a more detailed explanation a few days later
- Make information available about where the family can get help and support, with the names and addresses of outside agencies, including bereavement counselling and self-help groups
- Less educated patients and relatives often ask for more information than people who have had more education. This may be because they have less access to information or fewer skills to access it
- Summarise what has been said and consider a written follow-up. You may want to suggest tape-recording the discussion so that the relative or patient can listen to the explanations again, in their own time
- Use simple language; avoid euphemisms and medical jargon
- Probe to ensure that the person has understood. People do not always hear everything that is said after bad news has been delivered
- Decide on a clear method of recording what information each relative and patient has been told. This will enable you and your colleagues to check and support the information given and make it easier to judge who should receive further information, and when and at what level it should be given.

Recording the interview

The following information should be recorded during the interview:

- The key information that the family has been given
- What written information they have been given
- Whether or not they have been given a recording of the conversation
- If any medication has been prescribed
- If any tests have been organised
- If they have contact information about local support groups
- If they have a follow-up appointment for more information
- Who was present at the interview
- The time, place and duration of the interview
- Who is responsible for any further action required.

Discussions with bereavement care workers indicate that, ideally, a senior member of the medical staff should give bad news, as they would be in a position to answer any questions. It is helpful if a member of nursing staff can also be present and be available to discuss any areas of concern that the patient or relatives may have. Junior medical staff need training to ensure they understand how to convey bad news and the consequences of unthinking comments. When talking to Health Authority conveners and complaints staff it is very common to hear that a complainant has told staff that they complained about a general practitioner because someone in the Accident and Emergency Department had said, 'If the GP had referred the patient earlier they could have saved them'. This is sometimes said by more junior members of staff as a way of coping with a death by transferring responsibility to someone else. What they are really saying is, 'It is not my fault your relative died, it is the GP's fault'.

Poor communication

Anyone who has had any experience of dealing with complaints will often say that the key to preventing complaints is communication. Communication may be verbal, non-verbal or written and may be staff-to-staff, staff-to-patient or relative, or relative-to-relative. Complaints are often initiated by what appears to be an insignificant incident but this is often the final straw in a series of 'little incidents'.

The following points should be considered when communicating with patients or relatives:

- Be on the same level as the person you are talking to (e.g. do not stand if they are sitting or vice versa)
- Try to maintain eye contact
- Speak slowly and pause to allow the person to ask questions

secondary care

secondary care

2

- Observe the person for signs that they do not understand what you are telling them
- Be truthful but try to offer hope (for example, I am afraid you may not have long to live but we will not let you suffer any pain)
- Try to anticipate what the next question will be
- Do not rush the patient, especially if you are giving bad news.

Communication between staff members should also be clear and records should be kept of any interaction between staff concerning the care of the patient or the information given to relatives.

Non-verbal communication is as important as verbal communication when talking with patients and relatives. It is possible to tell if someone is angry or upset by observing them carefully. Eye contact is very important as it often indicates whether or not someone is being truthful; this is as true for the person giving the information as for the person receiving it. By observing the person you are communicating with it is possible to tell how the information that you are giving is being received and therefore whether an adjustment should be made. If, for example, it becomes apparent that the person does not understand what they are being told, or that they do not accept what they are being told, then presenting the information in a different way may help them to understand or accept the situation.

Poor record keeping

One of the areas that is key to the successful answering of a complaint is accurate record keeping. It is acknowledged that the staff on the wards and in clinics are busy but records give a contemporaneous account of what actually happened. However, there is a tendency amongst some staff to think that if a situation is unchanged or that tests are negative there is no need to record the information.

Telephone conversations should be recorded together with the date, time and the names of the parties involved in the conversation. This is especially important when talking to relatives who live some distance away, particularly if the patient is elderly or terminally ill. If a number of relatives are in contact with the hospital, a record should be kept of what information has been given to each relative. Anyone investigating a complaint should be able to follow through exactly what has happened to the patient with regard to treatment and action as a result of tests. Dates and times of events become very important and, if they are included, they can significantly speed up the time taken to investigate and therefore respond to a complainant. Experience shows that complainants who receive prompt and full responses are less likely to continue with their complaint.

Missed or late diagnosis

There are occasions when a diagnosis is missed, or when it takes a long time to obtain a definitive diagnosis. Unfortunately, there is a perception amongst the general public that the medical professions can diagnose and cure all ills. If a diagnosis has been missed it is important to explain to the patient how the diagnosis would normally be arrived at. Then an explanation should be given as to why the normal diagnosis was not possible earlier. This could be because another condition was masking the symptoms or because no signs and symptoms were present. If it takes a long time to find out what is wrong with the patient they should be informed why it is taking so long and reassured that everything is being done to find out what is wrong with them.

Poor complaint handling

A swift, full and accurate explanation will more often than not resolve a complaint, but the converse can also occur. Therefore, it is not surprising to note that complainants who progress to an Independent Review Panel often complain about the way their complaint has been handled. There are occasions when a lot of work and effort is put into handling a complaint but it appears to be impossible to satisfy the complainant. Patients who may fall into this category are those who have suffered a sudden bereavement or have mental health problems. Conversely, it may be that although the staff have done a lot of work they have not actually addressed the complainant's concerns or they have used jargon or terminology that is not understood by the complainant.

Other potential areas of complaint

The following are examples of incidents that could trigger a complaint if not handled correctly. Therefore it follows that if they are handled correctly the number of complaints may well reduce.

Being kept waiting

Patients who have arrived for a 9.00 a.m. appointment may be kept waiting without any explanation. For example, some clinics book patient appointments in blocks of five at half-hour intervals. This means that, if the clinic starts on time, at least four patients will be kept waiting. The argument is that it is important that the consultant is not kept waiting and anyway a percentage of patients do not attend for their appointments. This practice is not acceptable and patients should be booked in at realistic intervals. The appointment card should state the date and time of the appointment, where the patient has to attend and the action to take if they are unable to attend. The card should contain full details of who to contact, their telephone number, extension number and when they are available to take calls. Patients will not inform departments if they are unable to attend if it is not clear how to inform the department and who they should contact.

Patients may have been given correct appointment times but the clinic may be running late. In this instance, the staff should inform patients about the delay as soon as they arrive, and the reason for it, and apologise for the fact that they will be kept waiting. If the delay is lengthy (over an hour) the staff should consider suggesting that the patient goes away and returns later or, in some instances, offer another appointment. Staff need to remember that patients also have commitments, they may have to collect children from school, return to work, or return home to look after an elderly relative. The vast majority of patients will be happy to wait if the reason for any delay is explained as soon as they arrive.

People coming later and being seen first

Although staff understand the running of a hospital, patients do not always understand it. If a waiting area services several clinics, or if several staff are working in a clinic, it is worth taking time to explain to patients who they will be seeing and that there are several clinics running.

It is always worth checking if patients complain about being kept waiting. In one instance, some patients had been waiting well over an hour to see a consultant, although patients arriving later were being seen almost at once. Patients started to complain but were told that they were being seen in order. It eventually emerged that a member of staff was collecting appointment cards from patients and placing the new cards on the top of the pile rather than the bottom. The earlier patients were therefore getting further down the queue whilst the later patients were being seen at once. This was in spite of the fact that patients had been complaining and that there were written appointments.

Dealing with the next of kin

It is important to identify clearly who is the patient's next of kin. Once they have been identified, staff should ensure that if relatives are communicated with it is via this person. If the nominated next of kin lives a distance away from the Trust, day-to-day communication may well take place with a relative who lives nearby. If this is the case, steps should be taken to ensure that the identified next of kin is aware that a nearby relative is communicating with the Trust. It is easy for staff to presume that the two relatives will communicate with each other but this is not always the case. In these instances, record keeping becomes even more important as staff need to record what information was passed on to which relative and whether or not it was agreed that the relative would pass the information on.

Dealing with different relatives

Care should also be taken if a patient has a number of relatives who attend the Trust on a regular basis but at different times. In this scenario there is a danger that different people will give different relatives different pieces of information. As a result, each of the relatives may have part of the whole story but no one has the full picture. For example, two brothers had had a discussion with a consultant who informed them that he thought that their elderly mother had terminal cancer. He advised them that due to her physical condition it was, in his opinion, not advisable to do an operation to confirm the diagnosis, as he did not feel that she was fit enough for the anaesthetic. The brothers therefore agreed that no active treatment would be commenced with regard to the cancer but that general care and pain relief would be offered. After the mother's death the family complained about her care. At the subsequent Independent Review Panel it became apparent that although the conversation was recorded in the medical records and the brothers stated that they remembered the conversation and agreed that the record was accurate, the sister was not aware that the conversation had taken place, nor that there had been an initial diagnosis of cancer. Throughout the mother's stay in hospital all the family had visited on a regular basis and the staff had presumed that the brothers had discussed their mother's condition with their sister.

Being unable to get through on the telephone

Staff often complain that patients do not inform them when they are unable to keep a hospital appointment. But how often do the staff check the information printed on appointment cards and letters? These should be checked on a regular basis to make sure that the following information is accurate:

- The hospital telephone number, including STD code
- The ward/clinic name and extension number or direct dial number
- The name of the clinic/ward/consultant
- The times staff are available to take calls
- An out-of-hours telephone number where messages can be left
- Whether patients can make contact via fax or e-mail.

If staff are not available to take calls is there an answer phone/voice mail system, or can the phone be diverted so that messages can be left? Patients who are unable to get through because the telephone is constantly engaged,

2

secondary care

or rings but isn't answered may not bother to ring back or will become irritated with the lack of response. Increasingly, patients have access to alternative means of communication but how often are e-mail addresses and fax numbers made available to patients?

Patients not being given information

Trusts are becoming much better at sending out patient information but, again, how often is the information checked to make sure that it is accurate? Staff are familiar with ward routines but it may be the patient's first ever visit to a hospital. Sending patients a list of information about items that they need to bring with them and then telling them off for not bringing something that was not on the list does not lead to good patient–staff relations. For example, not informing patients that they should bring in a urine sample, or asking them to bring in a sample with no indication of the size of the sample or the type of container to use, is unhelpful and the lack of information could embarrass the patient.

Being given incorrect information

There will be occasions when patients or relatives are given incorrect information. If this happers then it is important that the error is acknowledged, corrected and an apology given as soon as possible. For example, a relative rang up to ask how her father was. The charge nurse informed her that her father was sitting up in bed, his condition was improving and that they were anticipating that he could be discharged at the weekend. Unfortunately, that evening he collapsed and the family were sent for, as the staff did not feel he would survive. When the daughter entered the ward the charge nurse approached her and apologised that the information she had been given earlier had been inaccurate. The charge nurse explained that he had acted in good faith but acknowledged how distressing the second telephone call must have been for the family. The relative later said that if the charge nurse had not approached the family they would probably have brought a complaint against the hospital.

Car parking

The lack of parking or the increasing trend of charging for hospital car parking places is tending to give rise to complaints. If charges are made or if there is a problem with car parking then this should be indicated on any appointment letter, with alternative options given. If the money from the car park is directly used by the Trust to improve patient services, notices to this effect at the payment points can help to inform patients and relatives.

Poor signposting

It is clear that there is a general issue about the quality of signposting. The frustration of not being able to find the correct car park, followed by the correct entrance and then the correct department is very sobering. Maps of the site can be helpful but only if they indicate where you are and if there is a clear feature that can easily be seen from that point. Once inside the building, frequent signposting is required, or the use of coloured lines or symbols, to help people find their way around the hospital.

Failing to act on complaints

Surveys over the years have shown that complainants say that they do not wish the same thing to happen to anyone else and that is the reason that they complain. In view of this comment, wherever possible Trusts should evaluate the complaints received and take action to try to prevent a re-occurrence. Unfortunately, although some Trusts are very good at evaluating complaints, they fail to take the next step of changing practice. One of the most constant themes running through complaints is the lack of communication. For example, if someone complains that they were not given a full explanation of the effects of a procedure, ideally the Trust should:

- See if written information is usually given out
- If there is no written information, consider whether this would be useful
- If written information is available, evaluate the content
- Consider involving groups like the CHC to evaluate the written material
- If the complaint covers only one area, check that it is not equally valid in other areas
- Finally, inform the complainant of any changes in procedure that have resulted from the complaint.

STAFF INVOLVEMENT

There will always be complaints in the NHS and it will not be possible to prevent all of them. But staff can go a long way in improving the way services are delivered to patients. A mechanism should be in place to enable staff to take note of and act on comments that are made by patients and relatives in a way that results in action being taken. If someone says, 'I had difficulty with the stairs' it is not sufficient to say, 'You could have used the lift'. If the person had difficulty they probably did not know that there was a lift, therefore are extra signs needed on the stairs to indicate where the nearest lift is?

2

secondary care

New staff members are a source of valuable information as to how services can be improved. As they come from outside the Trust they will notice areas of difficulty in the lay out of notes or the design of wards, clinics, forms, etc. Areas for potential improvement can therefore often be easily identified by interviewing new staff a few weeks after they have been in post.

17

Local Resolution

The vast majority of complaints are resolved at Local Resolution. It is true that the quicker that complaints are addressed and dealt with, the more likelihood there is for the complainant to be satisfied. If the staff of the Trust are empowered to handle complaints then only the more complex issues may result in a written letter of complaint with the involvement of the complaints manager and the chief executive. As Chapter 16 dealt with the Prevention of Complaints, this chapter will concentrate on the efficient and effective handing of complaints.

RECEIVING COMPLAINTS ON THE WARD OR IN A DEPARTMENT

If a·member of staff is approached by a patient or relative who is expressing dissatisfaction with the way a service is being offered then, wherever possible, that member of staff should address the complaint. Bearing in mind the principles of the complaint procedure, the person should be given a full explanation, an apology if appropriate and, wherever possible, steps should be put in place to try to prevent the problem happening again. For example, if a patient complains that they are having difficulty attracting staff using their buzzer, the following steps could be taken:

- Check that the buzzer is working correctly
  If it is not:
- Apologise to the patient
- Put in place alternative ways of gaining attention

secondary care

2

- Report the fault
- Arrange for the fault to be fixed
- Tell the patient what you have done
- Record the action taken.
  If it is working:
- Apologise to the patient
- Find out why it is not being answered
- Explain to the patient what the problems are
- Try to address the problem
- Report the problem (if appropriate)
- Record the action taken.

The above example may appear time consuming on a busy ward but in reality it will take very little time to address and the recording of the incident will demonstrate that action has been taken. One of the main problems with complaints that eventually get to an Independent Review Panel is the lack of supporting paper work. The staff often tell the panel that they have done things but if there is no record of the conversation or action taken it is very difficult for the panel if there is a difference of opinion between the parties concerned.

Often, what appears on the surface to be a small complaint can grow out of all proportion in the later stages. The complainant feels frustrated that no one is taking them seriously and the staff feel that the complaint is taking up a disproportionate part of their time. Taking care in the early stages can often result in the saving of a lot of time if the complaint continues through the process.

Initial checks and confidentiality

If the complainant is not the patient, be careful to make sure that patient confidentiality is not breached when answering the complaint. It is only possible to discuss the clinical aspects of a patient's care with a third party with the patient's consent. If a patient states that they do not wish other people to discuss their condition then that must be adhered to. In such a case, it should be explained to the person complaining why it is not possible for you to answer the complaint and that the patient's wishes are paramount. Again, it is important that an outline of the conversation is recorded.

When to pass a complaint on

If a patient or relative comments to a junior member of staff, that member of staff should deal with the complaint only if they are capable of responding to it fully.

For example, if a patient complains that they have been waiting for a bed pan then the member of staff involved should be able to say why they have been kept waiting and to apologise for the delay. If, on the other hand, a patient complains that they wish to go home and feel that they are being kept in hospital unnecessarily, then this may well need to be passed on to a senior member of staff.

The junior member of staff should explain to the patient why they are unable to respond. They should also tell the patient the name of the person they will be speaking to about their complaint. They then need to pass the complaint on as quickly as possible to ensure that it is dealt with speedily.

Complaints records and follow-up action

By keeping a record of all incidents that occur on the ward, any problems associated with the smooth running of the ward can easily be identified. This can only happen if the records are reviewed at regular intervals and action is taken. On the surface it may not appear to be important that relatives are complaining that there is nowhere for them to sit when visiting the patient. However, if this happens to a number of relatives visiting a number of patients, then action needs to be taken. In the above example, there may be several explanations each requiring alternative solutions. For example, insufficient chairs may be available because:

- There is a lack of chairs!
- There are sufficient chairs, but they are in another area of the ward
- Some patients are having large numbers of visitors
- Large numbers of visitors tend to arrive at the same time
- The majority of visitors arrive when the patients are in bed rather than in a day room.

Solutions to the above could include:

- Moving chairs from another ward or patient area
- Buying more chairs
- Asking a patients' organisation to buy more chairs
- Restricting visitors to a realistic number
- Seeing if the ward routine could be changed to make better use of the day room
- Seeing if visitors could be encouraged to attend at different times.

Reviewing and acting on complaints should hopefully reduce the number of complaints, in addition, the quality of a patient's stay in hospital should be improved.

THE COMPLAINTS DEPARTMENT

Written complaints are usually addressed to the chief executive but are handled by a Complaints Department. On the receipt of a written complaint the following questions should be asked before any action is taken.

- Is it appropriate for the NHS complaints procedure?
- Is consent required?
- Is access to medical records required?
- Is it a mixed sector complaint?
- Is the complaint out of time?
- Has disciplinary or legal action commenced?

Is it appropriate for the NHS complaints procedure?

The NHS complaints procedure is designed to deal with complaints about the provision of services at a hospital, including transport and the pathology service.

Problems arise if issues not covered under the NHS complaints procedure are dealt with under that procedure. Items that should not be dealt with include:

- Allegations of assault or fraud, as these are police matters and are therefore subject to their procedures
- Matters that are normally dealt with by other agencies, for example, noise from a residential home (which would be dealt with by the local authority's Environmental Health Department)
- The review procedure for continuing care, which is not subject to the complaints procedure.

It is important to refer these complaints to the appropriate agency as soon as possible. The NHS complaints procedure covers any complaint relating to the Trust's private beds but not medical care provided by a consultant outside their NHS contract. NHS work undertaken in private hospitals but contracted for and paid for by the NHS comes under the complaints procedure providing that the contractual agreement covers the action taken in the case of a complaint arising from the treatment.

Is consent required?

If the complainant is not the patient then written consent will usually be required for the person to pursue the complaint on the patient's behalf. If the patient is a minor or is unable to give consent then it is advisable to seek expert advice, as each case will rest on its own merit.

If the patient has died it rests with the complaints manager to decide whether the person acting on behalf of the patient is a suitable complainant. If they do not think they are a suitable person they can either refuse to deal with the complaint or nominate someone else to act on the patient's behalf. This could occur if a patient has expressly stated that certain information must not be disclosed to a third party. In this case, the third party should not be able to gain access to the information even after the patient has died.

Is access to medical records required?

If a patient is complaining about treatment they have received and, in order to investigate the complaint the patient's clinical records would have to be examined, then technically their consent is not required. Unfortunately, patients do not always realise that non-medical staff will be looking at their records. The NHS guidance states that patients have a right to refuse to allow access to their medical records and, if this happens, it would not be possible to investigate the clinical aspect of a complaint. However, the question then needs to be asked that, if patients are not aware that their records need to be examined, how can they withhold consent?

Is it a mixed sector complaint?

A complaint that covers more than one Trust, covers primary and secondary care or involves Social Services would be classed as a mixed sector complaint. The guiding principle is that a person needs to complain only once and that it is up to the person receiving the complaint to pass the appropriate section of the complaint on to the other parties and co-ordinate the responses.

Is the complaint out of time?

Complaints should be made within 6 months of the date the incident occurred or within 6 months of the time that it came to the complainant's notice, providing no more than 12 months have elapsed from the original incident. If a complaint is received after the time specified it is up to the complaints manager to decide whether it would have been unreasonable for the complaint to be made earlier and that it is still possible to investigate the complaint properly.

It must be remembered that once a complaint has been accepted under the NHS complaints procedure then the complainant has the right to continue through the whole process. Staff should therefore ensure that it is possible to investigate a complaint fully before it is accepted. It is possible to tell people that a complaint is out of time and explain that it cannot be accepted under the complaints procedure but to agree that the Trust will endeavour to answer any questions. It would be necessary then to explain the limitations of any investigation and why it would not be possible to give a full explanation. For example, this could happen if a ward had been closed or the staff had left the area.

2

secondary care

Has disciplinary or legal action commenced?

If it is felt that a complaint is so serious that disciplinary action is required then the complaint should be referred for disciplinary action. If disciplinary action is taken then that aspect of the complaint cannot be investigated under the complaints procedure. Any information that has been accumulated during the initial investigation can be passed on to the persons initiating the disciplinary action. The complainant will therefore be told that disciplinary action has been taken. If it is decided that disciplinary action is not going to be taken then the complaint should be investigated under the complaints procedure and the complainant informed accordingly.

If the complainant states that they intend to take legal action then the complaints procedure should stop. Some Trusts have presumed that a letter from a solicitor indicates that the complainant is taking legal action; this is not necessarily the case and the complaints manager should contact the solicitor concerned and ask if their client is taking legal action against the Trust. This should clarify the situation.

ACKNOWLEDGEMENT LETTER

Any written complaint should be acknowledged by the Trust within two working days of receipt of the complaint. This acknowledgement letter should inform the complainant – either in the body of the letter or by way of a complaints leaflet – of the following:

- The options open to the complainant under Local Resolution (written response, meeting)
- Where they can get help and advice (for example the CHC)
- When the complainant can expect a reply (within 20 days)
- The options available if the complainant remains dissatisfied after Local Resolution
- Details of a contact person
- Details of the Ombudsman.

THE INVESTIGATION

Once a complaint has been received and accepted then an investigation needs to be undertaken. This is often done by a senior member of staff in the ward or department concerned. One of the major problems associated with complaints investigation is the time involved in doing a thorough job but, as stated earlier, time taken at this stage can save more time later. In fact, a thorough investigation and response, handled in an open and honest way, will often resolve the complaint.

Problems arise when people investigating the complaint do not speak to the staff involved in the complaint. Instead the investigators say what they thought would have happened, forgetting that what may be a routine occurrence for them is often a once-in-a-lifetime experience for the patient or relative.

Conducting an investigation

The steps to be followed when conducting an investigation are listed below:

• Collect the relevant papers
• Evaluate the letter of complaint
• Interview the staff concerned
• Prepare a written response.

Collect the relevant papers

Before embarking on an investigation, collect together: the letter of complaint, any other complaints correspondence, the appropriate section of the patient's records and any other supporting information. Examples could include, appointment sheets, theatre lists, patient information sheets, consent forms, local protocols.

Evaluate the letter of complaint

If possible, try to list the complaints as identified by the complainant. This will enable a check to be made to ensure that all the issues have been fully addressed. Identify which staff were involved with the patient at the time of the complaint and make arrangements to interview each of the staff involved.

Also try to identify what the person wants:

• Is it to improve the service for others?
• Has something gone wrong and they wish to know why it happened?
• Is it to understand what has happened to a relative?
• Could they be having difficulty in coming to terms with the loss of a loved one?

It is very possible that the complaint identifies ways in which the service could be improved:

• Is it within your remit to bring about such improvements?
• Do more senior staff need to become involved?
• Could other areas benefit from the improvement?
• How could you disseminate any lessons learnt?

Interview the staff concerned

Many staff are very deeply affected by complaints; it is not unusual for staff to recall complaints that happened many years previously. When reading one person's view of a situation it is very easy to presume that something very serious happened, only to find that the picture changes completely when you read the other side of the story. It is therefore vital to keep an open mind and to treat staff sensitively. Interviews should be conducted in private and not in the middle of an open ward or department. Remind staff that you are trying to establish what happened and wish to hear their version of events. Ask if they remember the patient and the incident referred to in the complaint and do not be surprised if they do not. Make sure that the appropriate records are available and allow the staff to remind themselves by reading the records. If the staff do not remember and the information they give is from the records only, make sure that this is very clear in your report. The staff may not remember but the complainant will, and will therefore notice any errors and draw conclusions from those errors, which may or may not be appropriate.

Try to take each of the points raised in the complaint in turn. If the information given is backed up by written records, say so and, where possible, quote directly from the records. If there are omissions in the records it is important to say why the information was not recorded.

Encourage the staff to make a written statement of their recollection of the events in question and ask them to date and sign it. They will find this useful if further questions arise.

Advise the staff where they can get help and support, sometimes staff become very upset and this can affect their work.

Prepare a written response

Depending on Trust policy, the response will either be sent with a covering letter from the chief executive or it will be incorporated into a letter from the chief executive. The most effective way of responding is to list all the areas of concern, using each one as a heading, and to provide the response under each heading. In this way it is very easy to check the reply by making sure that:

- All areas of concern have been covered
- All medical terms have been explained
- A lay person could understand the response
- Background information is supplied to help the complainant to understand what happened
- An apology is included, if it is appropriate
- If something has gone wrong, the steps taken to try and prevent it happening again have been included
- The information provided is accurate and complete
- If information is based on written records the records used are clearly identified

- If the staff do not remember an incident, it is stated that they do not remember and an explanation of what is normal practice is included
- The offer of a meeting is made, if appropriate
- Condolences are offered if the patient has died.

Informal meetings

Following the written response, a complainant may wish to speak either to the staff involved in the complaint or to their line manager. Who meets with the staff will be decided by the Trust and will depend on the level and seniority of the person involved in the complaint. For example, the ward leader may become involved if the complaint concerns a junior nurse, or a consultant if the complaint is about a house officer.

The complaints manager will often arrange the meeting and will attend to informally chair the meeting and to take minutes of the proceedings. The following factors should be taken into account when a meeting is being organised:

- Who should attend
- The organisation of the room
- Paperwork required
- Minute taking
- Checking the minutes
- The use of external clinicians
- The use of lay conciliators.

Who should attend

The complainant will wish to attend the meeting but the complaints manager needs to decided who can accompany them to the meeting. Other relatives are often involved in a complaint and the complainant may wish to bring a CHC representative with them. On balance, it is often better to allow all the relatives who wish to attend to come with the complainant. It is often not clear from the correspondence who the main complainant is and, in some instances, the person writing the letter of complaint may be doing so on behalf of someone else.

If large numbers of relatives are attending, it is better, if possible, to ask if they can agree that one person acts as the spokesperson for the group, although flexibility will be needed on behalf of the Trust. The CHC often attends these meetings but, again, it is better if the complainant can be encouraged to ask their own questions rather than allowing the CHC officer to take the lead. It must be remembered that it is the complainant's complaint and they are the only person that truly knows what their concerns are. In some instances it is only at a meeting that the true areas of concern emerge.

secondary care

secondary care

2

If the complaint involves a number of members of Trust staff it is better that they do not all attend the meeting at the same time. To walk into a room and be presented with a row of senior staff, along with the complaints manager and a secretary, can be very intimidating for a complainant. It can also give rise to comments that 'they were ganging up on me' or that the staff were 'sticking together'.

A more acceptable approach is for the complainant to meet initially with the complaints manager and the person who is taking the minutes of the meeting. The staff are then invited to attend one at a time, each answering the concerns of the complainant. When a member of staff has completed their discussions they telephone the next member of staff and ask them to attend the meeting. This approach gives the complainant time to gather their thoughts between seeing individual members of staff. It also means that the staff make much more effective use of their time.

The organisation of the room

Any meeting under Local Resolution should be as informal as possible. The use of low chairs and coffee tables may well be appropriate as every effort should be made to ensure that the meeting does not become confrontational. The offer of tea or coffee and the availability of drinking water can also help. A box of tissues is advisable, especially in cases of bereavement – far better to have a box in the room than to have to go off and hunt for one if someone becomes upset. If the meeting can take place in a non-patient area of the hospital this can often be more acceptable to the complainant, especially in cases of bereavement.

If tables are used, try to make sure that everyone sits round the same table and, wherever possible, select a room that is neither too large nor too small. The use of an adjacent office where the CHC officer can talk to the complainant before and after the meeting is often appreciated. This arrangement can often provide initial feedback on the success of the meeting, although experience shows that it is usually very clear whether the complainant has been satisfied by the meeting.

Paperwork required

Wherever possible, the complaints file, the copy of the original letter of complaint and the written response should be available at the meeting. If the response letter has listed the complaints, it makes the organisation of the meeting much easier if this used as a basis for discussions. Prior to the meeting the complaints manager can discuss with the complainant which areas of the response they are still unhappy with and also which areas of the response they do not understand or do not agree with. This will focus the discussions and make sure that the complainant's concerns are answered fully.

secondary care

The appropriate, original clinical records and any other supporting documentation should also be available at the meeting. This will enable the clinical staff to discuss the contents of the records with the complainant if required.

Minute taking

It is important to keep a record of the meeting, stating who attended, the date and time. Although this does not need to be a verbatim report it is helpful if any explanations are noted under the appropriate areas of concern. When taking minutes of the meeting it should be remembered that if the complainant requests an Independent Review Panel they have to state what areas remain outstanding and why they remain dissatisfied. After taking clinical advice the convener and the lay chair go through the correspondence (including the minutes of any meetings) and decide whether a full explanation has been given. If the minutes of the meeting state, 'The consultant answered the issues raised about the surgery' the convener and lay chair would not know what explanation was given or whether or not it was full. They would therefore have to decide whether to return the complaint to Local Resolution or grant an Independent Review Panel. If, on the other hand, the minutes detailed what the surgeon had said, they could decide that a full explanation had been given and nothing further could be added by granting an Independent Review Panel and therefore refuse the request.

Checking the minutes

It is advisable for copies of the minutes of the meeting to be sent to the staff involved so that they can confirm their accuracy. Once the staff have checked the minutes they can then be sent to the complainant with a request that they notify the Trust if there are any corrections to be made. This ensures that the complainant has a record of the discussion that took place. Often, especially if they are upset, people do not remember all that was said at meetings, and minutes that they can re-read will help them to discuss the meeting more constructively with their relatives or the CHC. It also means that there is a full record on file for the convener to access if necessary. If the minutes are not sent to the complainant they could say that certain issues were not discussed. By asking them to agree the minutes the Trust is in a position to demonstrate that the issues either had or had not been discussed.

The use of external clinicians

As the approach used for Local Resolution is up to the Trust involved, there may be instances when an external clinical opinion may assist in resolving

secondary care

2

a complaint. If, for example, the patient feels that the Trust is covering up, or not providing all the information available, a review by an external person may help to resolve the complaint. The provision of a report by an independent consultant who provides an explanation for the clinical decisions taken and confirms that they were taken in line with current practice may help to reassure the complainant. If, on the other hand, the independent clinician raises areas of concern then the Trust has an opportunity to address these concerns and inform the complainant of the action that has been taken. It is not suggested that this is done as a matter of routine but there are occasions when this approach can provide a way through a particularly difficult complaint.

The use of lay conciliators

All Health Authorities have to appoint lay conciliators, who are used widely in primary care but not as extensively by Trusts, as the complaints manager often has the expertise to handle complaints and investigate fully. However, there are several instances when an independent lay conciliator can help to resolve a complaint. If the complainant refuses to meet with anyone in the Trust and will not discuss their concerns, a conciliator can act as an 'honest broker'. They can meet with the complainant and then go and talk to the staff involved and provide a response. This is often useful if the complainant lives a long way away from the Trust.

In cases of sudden bereavement, for example, connected with the loss of a child or young person, the parents may direct their anger at the Trust where the child died. They may feel that the Trust was responsible for the death of the child and therefore will not believe any information that comes from the Trust. If all parties are in agreement, a meeting with the parents and an independent clinician, facilitated by a lay conciliator, may provide the parents with some of the explanations and reassurances they need. In order to successfully resolve the complaint, the medical records should be available at the meeting and the clinician concerned will need to be familiar with the case.

A sudden death caused by septicaemia following meningitis would be an example of the type of case that may well benefit from this approach. The general public often does not realise that there are several types of meningitis, they want to know why a vaccination was not offered or, if their child had had a vaccination, why it did not work. They are unable to comprehend why their child died so quickly and may feel guilty that they did not act sooner. It is very difficult to provide answers to the above questions in writing. A discussion with explanations can often help, although it can never be said that the parents will be truly satisfied with any explanation given to them.

2

THE CHIEF EXECUTIVE'S RESPONSE

Suggested format for the response letter

Wherever possible, the complaints should be listed with the appropriate response under each complaint. Some chief executives like the response to be incorporated in the body of a letter. Others attach a report of the investigation to the covering letter. The latter has the advantage of using headings and lists in a 'report format', thus reducing the reading age of the letter and making it easier to read. It also means that it is easier to ensure that all aspects of the complaint have been answered. The disadvantage is that the report could become separated from the letter and, if this technique is used, the covering letter should clearly state that a report is attached and give the report's title. It is also helpful if the report is dated.

The complainant's rights

The complainant has a right to request an Independent Review Panel within 28 days of the end of Local Resolution. It is therefore important that the last letter advises the complainant of these rights.

The chief executive must send the final letter of Local Resolution. One of the biggest problems is that it is very difficult to gauge which is the final letter. Local Resolution in Trusts often goes through several stages, which may include:

- A written response
- A meeting with the staff concerned
- A meeting with a senior member of staff (either from the Trust or a neighbouring Trust)
- The use of lay conciliation.

If the complainant has received a complaints leaflet, or if the acknowledgement letter outlines the complaints procedure, the original response letter could include a statement along the lines of:

I (the chief executive) have tried to give you a full response to your concerns. If, however, you have further questions or remain dissatisfied, please contact ... within 28 days of this letter. He/she will explain the options open to you under the NHS complaints procedure.

The complainant should be given a contact address and telephone number. If they contact the Trust they could then be offered a further written response, a meeting, or details of how to contact the convener, depending on the stage that the complaint has reached.

Technically, once a complaint has been accepted under the complaints procedure, if the 'last letter' does not give the complainant 28 days to request on Independent Review Panel, then the complaint remains open.

secondary care

2

Therefore, if a complainant came back 1 year later they would not be 'out of time' as Local Resolution would be still in progress.

In case the complainant wishes to request an Independent Review Panel, they should be advised:

- How to contact the convener
- Of the 28-day time limit for making the request
- Where they can get help and assistance
- That they need to state what issues remain outstanding from Local Resolution
- That they need to say why they remain dissatisfied.

The Convening Decision

If a complainant writes requesting an Independent Review Panel, the complaint is dealt with by the Trust convener in consultation with an independent lay chair. In the case of clinical complaints the convener will need to take clinical advice, usually from a member of the Trust staff.

THE COMPLAINTS MANAGER

The complaints manager is responsible for providing the administrative support for the Convening Decision. All parties will require a copy of all correspondence between the complainant and the Trust, along with the minutes of any meetings that have taken place and the file notes of any conversations. It is helpful to all concerned if the papers are put in date order and are numbered before being photocopied. In addition, the clinical advisor will require copies of the relevant medical records e.g. a nurse will require the nursing records; a physiotherapist, the physiotherapy records and a consultant the medical records.

2

secondary care

The complaints manager will also be responsible for making sure that:

- The initial checks and associated paper work have been completed
- Acknowledgement letters are sent out (the time limit is 2 days for the acknowledgement by the convener)
- The identification and the appointment of the lay chair takes place at the earliest possible stage
- The outstanding issues have been identified
- The time limit of 20 days for the Convening Decision is being adhered to
- All parties are informed of the reason for the delay if the time limits are not going to be met
- The papers are returned at the end of the Convening Decision and are stored separately from the patient records
- The expenses forms are completed and processed promptly.

THE INITIAL CHECKS
Knowledge of the parties

It is important to check that the complainant is not known to the convener or other members of the team before the papers are sent out. It is not acceptable to send out the papers and then ask the question.

Time limits

As the complainant should make the request for an Independent Review Panel within 28 calendar days of the final letter of Local Resolution, a check should be made on the dates of both letters. If the request is made outside the 28-day limit, it is up to the convener to decide whether or not it would have been unreasonable for the complainant to make the request within the time scales. It is possible for the time scales to be extended, for example, if the complainant has been ill and therefore unable to meet the 28-day deadline. In addition, the convener should decide whether or not it would still be possible to investigate the complaint properly.

Outstanding issues

It is very clear in the directions that the complainant needs to identify, in writing, the issues that remain outstanding from Local Resolution and why they remain dissatisfied. Therefore, if the initial request from the complainant does not explain this, the convener should write to the complainant advising them that these statements are necessary if their request is to be considered. It is helpful if the complainant can be advised of the names, addresses and telephone numbers of people who could assist them, for example, the local CHC or the Citizen's Advice Bureau. In addition, the complainant should be advised of a date by which the Trust would expect to hear from them, as one of the principles behind the complaints system is that complaints should be dealt with as quickly as possible. A reasonable time to expect a response would be in the order of 10 working days.

If the complainant writes back and still fails to identify the outstanding issues and why they remain dissatisfied, it is possible for the convener or a member of staff to list all the issues. The list is then sent to the complainant with a request that they confirm that all the issues have been covered. It will make the role of the convener much easier if, when writing this letter, the issues are presented in date order and are numbered. This ensures that all issues are covered in any subsequent correspondence. Again, it is helpful if the complainant can be advised of a date when the Trust would expect to hear from them.

THE APPOINTMENT OF PARTIES

The convener

The number of conveners appointed by a Trust will depend on the size of the Trust. Every Trust must appoint one non-executive to take on the role of the convener but additional associate conveners may also be appointed. If the convener is a non-executive director they do not receive extra payment for their role as convener and are indemnified for this role in the same way that they are indemnified for carrying out their role as non-executive directors.

Associated conveners can be reimbursed sessional fees, at the rate determined by the Trust, in addition to travel and out-of-pocket expenses. Associate conveners should also be indemnified by the Trust for their work as an associate convener.

When a new convener is appointed, the appropriate Regional Office should be advised of the appointment.

The lay chair

The appropriate Regional Office is responsible for recruiting and training the lay chairs. These are people who are not involved with the Trust and provide the independent element to the Convening Decision process.

When a request for an Independent Review Panel is received, a request is made to the Regional Office for a lay chair. The regional officers nominate a lay chair and, in doing so, try to ensure that, wherever possible, the lay chair has not been involved with a previous Independent Review request at that Trust. This is done in order to ensure that the independence

2

secondary care

of the lay chair is maintained and that the lay chair does not get too involved with a Trust.

Once the name of the lay chair is known, and after the check is made to ensure that they do not know the parties concerned, a formal letter of appointment is sent out from the Trust.

As from this point the lay chair is working for the Trust the letter of appointment should include the following:

- A confidentiality statement
- Confirmation of indemnity cover
- Details of travel, subsistence and financial loss allowance payable
- Details of how to claim for incidental expenses (postage and telephone costs)
- Instructions about the return of papers
- Details of how to contact the convener
- A contact name at the Trust with an address, the telephone and fax numbers and an e-mail address.

A confidentiality statement

The lay chair will see the letters and minutes of any meetings that have taken place in the course of the investigation of the complaint. Some of the papers may contain details about the patient's medical condition. With the advent of the Caldicott Guardians there is a very high level of importance attached to confidentiality and Trusts have a duty of care to ensure that any information concerning patients is handled correctly.

To ensure that people act appropriately they should be reminded of the importance of:

- Confidentiality
- The correct storage of papers
- Not discussing the complaint to any third party in any way that the patient can be identified.

Confirmation of indemnity cover

As the lay chair will be working for the Trust when they take part in the Convening Decision they should be indemnified by the Trust for their work. The Trust's own insurers will add lay chairs to the cover but a check should be made to make sure that this has happened.

Details of travel, subsistence and financial loss allowance payable

The Department of Health produces guidance on these rates. Lay chairs cannot be paid for the work they undertake but they are able to claim demonstrable loss of earnings. Therefore, if a lay chair took time off from work and, as a result, their salary was reduced, they could claim back that loss. There is a problem around the area of self-employment as the payment is for actual, rather than potential, loss of earnings. It is advisable that the Trust formulates a policy for payment including possibly a maximum daily rate that they are prepared to reimburse.

Details of how to claim for incidental expenses

The Trust should be prepared to reimburse the cost of postage and telephone calls. The lay chair should be told the rates payable and sent a claim form with information concerning when the form should be returned and to whom.

Instructions about the return of papers

As has already been mentioned, the Trust has a duty of care to make sure that patient information does not get into the public domain. The Department of Health has stated that complaint papers should be stored for the same length of time as patient's records. Therefore, if all records are returned to the Trust on the completion of the Convening Decision, a full set of records can be stored. Personal notes made by the lay chair can be placed in an envelope and stored with the records so that they can be retrieved at a later date if required. It is not satisfactory for the lay chair, or anyone else involved in the process, to destroy any of the records – how would the Trust know if they had been destroyed correctly? In one instance, a lay chair said that they always burnt papers, which on the face of it sounded appropriate. However, on further questioning it turned out that what they actually did was place the papers in a plastic sack and take them to the local refuse tip for incineration. It had not occurred to them that this course of action made it possible for a third person to see the documents before incineration.

Contact details

It can save much time and effort if full contact details are supplied at the beginning of the process. The use of e-mail is increasing and many lay chairs also have fax facilities available to them. Having a named person who can be contacted at the Trust ensures that the process can be efficiently handled, hopefully within the 20 working days allocated to the Convening Decision.

The clinical advisors

If the complaint contains a clinical element then the convener must take clinical advice. It is possible for the convener to use clinicians working in the Trust, providing they have not been involved in any aspect of the Local Resolution process. The emphasis has been placed on conveners taking appropriate clinical advice and, in the case of the more complex complaints, more than one clinical advisor may be required. If, for example, the complaint involved a nurse, a gynaecologist and a physiotherapist, clinical advice would have to be taken from three specialists.

The medical or nursing director could give advice to the convener or advise on the most appropriate departmental head to do so. It is not possible, for example, for the medical director to give advice if they had been involved in Local Resolution. If the staff of the Trust are unable to give clinical advice then the Regional Office should be asked for the name of a person who is able to advise the convener.

THE PRINCIPLES BEHIND THE CONVENING DECISION

The aim of the Convening Decision is for the convener, in conjunction with the lay chair to evaluate whether or not the aims of the complaints procedure have been met. Namely:

1. Has a full and complete explanation, of what happened and why, been given in terminology that the complainant can understand?

2. Has an apology been given if there was an error or omission on behalf of the staff of the Trust?

3. If there was an error or omission, has information been given about the action that the Trust has or is proposing to take to try and prevent it happening again?

In addition, can any further information be given to the complainant to help to resolve the complaint?

Independence versus impartiality

One of the criticisms levied at the Convening Decision is how can the convener, as a non-executive member of the Trust, be independent? It is important to realise that the convener is not independent of the Trust – they cannot be, as they are responsible for the actions of the Trust. What the convener *is* able to be is impartial. They should not 'take sides', nor should they write as if they are acting on behalf of the Trust. They should try to take as structured an approach as possible and should be able to demonstrate their impartiality by the way that they handle the decision-making process.

On the other hand, the lay chair *is* independent from the Trust. As has already been mentioned, the Regional Office tries to allocate a different lay chair for each Independent Review Panel request to maintain the independence.

secondary care

Criticism has also been levied at the process because the clinical advice is usually obtained from Trust staff. It is very clear that Trust staff can be used to advise the convener and criticism often comes from people who do not understand the aims behind the convening process. There is a perception that clinical advice is a means of obtaining a second opinion on a complaint, which is not the case.

Some of the misunderstandings have arisen due to the language and terminology used in some complaints leaflets and correspondence. When checking literature it may be useful to bear in mind the following points:

- It is *the convener*, not the independent convener
- The *convener is impartial*, not independent
- It is *the independent lay chair*
- The convener obtains *clinical advice* not independent clinical advice.

What is being evaluated?

The convener, the lay chair and the clinical advisor have copies of:

- The outstanding issues, as identified by or approved by the complainant
- All correspondence between the complainant and the Trust
- Any file notes of telephone conversations or other conversations
- Minutes of meetings that have taken place during the Local Resolution process.

In addition, the clinical advisor has copies of the appropriate medical or nursing records.

The convener, the lay chair and the clinical advisor look at each of the outstanding issues in turn. Their role is to evaluate whether or not the aims of the complaints procedure have been met for each of the issues that remain outstanding. If the aims have not been met the decision is whether more could be done at Local Resolution or if the only way to satisfy the complainant is to convene an Independent Review Panel.

The purpose of the Convening Decision is therefore not to pass judgement on the treatment but to evaluate the Local Resolution process. If an error has been made and has been acknowledged by the Trust, an apology given and the complainant told of the steps that have been taken to try to prevent it happening again, then no further action can be taken. As a result, any request for an Independent Review Panel should be refused.

AN OVERVIEW OF THE CONVENING DECISION

The role of the convener and the lay chair is to review the correspondence and file notes from Local Resolution and decide whether the aims of the complaints procedure have been met for each of the outstanding issues outlined by the complainant.

Should the parties be interviewed?

The guidance document produced by the NHS Executive suggests that the convener and lay chair may wish to interview the parties involved. However, in subsequent reports, the Ombudsman has criticised conveners for investigating complaints. Over the years it has become clear that, although technically the convener and the lay chair may talk to the complainant, this should be done only in very exceptional circumstances. If the complainant is unable to state what issues are outstanding it is better that they are advised where to go for help, for example, the CHC, rather than the convener becoming involved. Unfortunately, it is very difficult not to get drawn into a complaint if you have direct contact with a complainant, who may ask the convener such questions as:

- Do you think I have grounds for complaint?
- Don't you think I should have had the tests?
- Have you had many complaints about X?
- Lots of people I know have had the same complaint about X; don't you find he/she is always rude to patients?

By answering any of the above questions the convener will have been drawn into the complaint and runs the risk either of being accused of investigating the complaint or of not treating both parties equally. It could also be argued that if the convener talks to one of the parties they should also talk to the other party, thus becoming even more involved.

Some conveners (and lay chairs) have said that if only they could talk to the parties they could resolve the complaint. This may well be true but it is not their role. It is for the Trust staff in Local Resolution or the Independent Review Panel to resolve the complaint. On balance, it would therefore be advisable for conveners not to have direct contact with any of the parties involved in the complaint.

Taking clinical advice

When the NHS complaints procedure first came into being, many conveners met with the clinical advisors and discussed the complaint with them. The conveners argued that they needed to see the clinical records and to discuss the complaint in order to understand it. By taking this line they showed that they had misunderstood their role. If, after reading the letters of explanation sent out by the Trust to the complainant and looking at the minutes of meetings where explanations had been given, they failed to understand the complaint, then it would be reasonable to assume that the complainant would also misunderstand and probably explains why they had requested an Independent Review Panel. The convener's decision would then be where it was best to get the full explanation required, either in further Local Resolution or by convening an Independent Review Panel.

In addition, very little training has taken place for clinical advisors. In the past, many felt that their role was one of reviewing the whole of the case and commenting on whether or not the action taken had been appropriate. This is not their role under the current complaints procedure. A convener who asks specific questions in a letter, or uses a clinical advice form, will receive an appropriate and structured written response. This can then be passed directly to the lay chair, ensuring that both the convener and the lay chair have identical information available to them.

The medical records

As both the convener and the lay chair are lay people it is not necessary for them to have copies of the clinical records. It is for the clinical advisor to look at the clinical records to see if any additional information has not been passed on to the complainant and would help to address the outstanding issues.

An example would be if a complainant had complained about a delay in diagnosis. If the explanations given to the complainant stated that the clinicians were unable to confirm the diagnosis earlier and that the patient was given the diagnosis at the earliest possible time, the clinical advisor may suggest that the information given was correct but that it had omitted to give details of the number and type of tests given, all of which had negative results. The clinical advisor could recommend a meeting between the complainant and a clinician in order to explain which tests had been done and why it was not possible to make an earlier diagnosis.

How the decision is made

Working independently, the convener and the lay chair should take each of the outstanding issues in turn. They should look through the correspondence, minutes of meetings and the written clinical advice.

It is usual for the convener to telephone the lay chair. In simple complaints, involving only one or two outstanding issues, the decision can often be made at this stage. In more complex complaints, it may be necessary for the convener and the lay chair to meet.

It is essential that the convener does not try to influence the lay chair. The usual approach would be for them to discuss each outstanding issue in turn. The convener would ask for the lay chair's decision and reasons for the decision. If they are in agreement, they would move on to the next issue. If there is disagreement, they could discuss the issue. The final decision rests with the convener.

A file note should be made of the discussion and a record placed in the complaints file.

Options available at the Convening Decision

Four options are available to the convener and the lay chair at the convening stage:

1. Refer back for further Local Resolution
2. Refuse the request for an Independent Review Panel
3. Agree to hold an Independent Review Panel
4. Ask the Trust whether disciplinary proceedings should be initiated.

It is possible to have a combination of the above options when dealing with each complaint. Following the decision, the convener would write to the complainant, the parties involved in the complaint and the Trust chief executive, advising them of the decision.

Refer back for further Local Resolution

This option would take place if it was felt that there was further action that could be taken under Local Resolution, or if a new complaint had emerged, in which case it would *have* to be referred back to Local Resolution. In this instance, the convener would write to all parties informing them of the decision, with suggestions for further action. These could include, for example, meetings, lay conciliation or explanations about particular aspects of the complaint. When wording this response, the convener should take care not to inadvertently make two decisions. For example:

I have decided to turn down your request for an Independent Review Panel as I have decided to refer your case back to Local Resolution

A better form of wording would be:

I have discussed your request for an Independent Review Panel with an independent lay chair and we have decided to refer your case back for further Local Resolution.

This second example offers only one option.

The convener is also required to advise the complainant that, if further Local Resolution does not resolve the complaint, they have a right to re-request an Independent Review Panel and that this should be done within 28 days of the final letter of Local Resolution.

Refuse the request for an Independent Review Panel

If all the aims of the complaints process have been met, or if no further action can be taken, the decision may be to refuse the request for an

secondary care

Independent Review Panel. This might occur if there was a complaint about manner and attitude and no-one else was present at the time of the incident. If one of the parties states that the other was rude, and the person accused denies being rude, it would be very difficult to add any further information as it is a case of one person's word against the other's. This would be especially true if the correspondence contained a statement apologising for the fact that the manner and attitude of the member of staff was felt by the patient to be unsatisfactory.

When refusing a request for an Independent Review Panel the convener should indicate where the outstanding issue had been answered. For example:

I note in the letter from the chief executive to you, dated 30 January, that the reason for the 3-hour delay in being seen in the out-patient clinic was because the consultant had to deal with an emergency that had arisen on the ward. After consulting with the independent lay chair we have decided that the explanation given to you in that letter was full and complete and we do not believe that any further information could be forthcoming from an Independent Review Panel. We have therefore decided to refuse your request for an Independent Review Panel on that point.

As the convener has refused the request for the Independent Review Panel it is necessary to include details of the complainant's right to contact the Ombudsman and his name, address and telephone number should therefore be included in the letter.

Agree to hold an Independent Review Panel

If the decision is to hold an Independent Review Panel then it is up to the convener to write the terms of reference for the panel. These are based on those outstanding issues that require further explanation. In view of the fact that the Independent Review Panel is not disciplinary, it is usual for the terms of reference to be open statements and time limited. For example:

To investigate Mrs X's stay in hospital from 3 to 9 August.

To evaluate the discharge arrangements made for Mr Y on 10 September.

Although it is the convener's role to write the terms of reference, the responsibility for the Independent Review Panel rests with the independent lay chair. It is therefore good practice check the wording of the terms of reference with the lay chair prior to sending them out.

The convener then writes to all parties advising them that a panel is being convened and giving the terms of reference for the panel.

Much discussion has taken place as to whether or not the terms of reference should be agreed with the complainant. Bearing in mind that they will be based on the outstanding issues as identified by the complainant, and that it is not possible to investigate any new issues at Independent Review Panel stage, the decision is one for the convener. The trend appears to be that, once agreed with the lay chair, the terms of reference are sent to the complainant with a request to notify the convener if there are any corrections or comments.

Ask the Trust whether disciplinary proceedings should be initiated?

If, at first sight, it appears that there are grounds for disciplinary action, the convener should ask the appropriate person in the Trust to decide whether to take disciplinary action. If part, or all, of the complaint is referred to disciplinary action, and it is agreed that disciplinary action is to take place, then the complainant should be advised that no further action will be taken under the complaints procedure with regard to that aspect of the complaint. Any aspect of the complaint not referred for disciplinary action is treated in the same way as a normal request for an Independent Review Panel.

If it is decided by the Trust that no disciplinary action will take place then the regulations state that 'a panel shall be appointed'.

IF THE COMPLAINANT DISAGREES WITH THE CONVENER'S DECISION

The complainant does not have a right to have an Independent Review Panel. If the complainant does not wish to go back to Local Resolution, that is their right but, once the Convening Decision has been made it should not be changed. Therefore, if the complainant chooses not to go back to Local Resolution then the complaints procedure stops. Providing that the convener's recommendations for further Local Resolution were reasonable then, if the complainant subsequently goes to the Ombudsman, they would be advised that he could not get involved as Local Resolution had not been completed.

If the complainant disagrees with the convener's decision not to convene a panel they have a right to go to the Ombudsman. If the Ombudsman feels that the correct process was not followed he may invite the convener to reconsider the decision. This could happen if, for example, the convener had not taken clinical advice. The convener would then go through the decision-making process again, taking clinical advice. The final decision may or may not be the same.

CORRESPONDENCE AT THE CONVENING STAGE

The following correspondence is usually sent out during the convening process:

- An initial acknowledgement letter from the complaints manager
- An appointment letter to the lay chair (as outlined on p. 171)

- An acknowledgement letter to the complainant from the convener (sent within 2 days)
- A letter from the convener to the complained against informing them of the outstanding issues identified by the complainant
- A letter from the convener to the clinical advisor(s) outlining the process
- A letter from the convener to the lay chair outlining the process
- A file note of the discussion that takes place between the convener and the lay chair
- A letter from the convener to the complainant giving information concerning the final decision
- A letter from the convener to any person complained against giving their final decision
- A letter to the chief executive.

Initial acknowledgement letter

Receipt of the initial letter requesting an Independent Review Panel should be acknowledged by the Trust. The acknowledgement letter would indicate that the request had been received and was being passed on to the convener, who would in turn acknowledge receipt of the request to the complainant.

Acknowledgement letter from the convener

This letter should be sent within two working days of the request being received by the convener. The type of information that may be included in the letter is:

- An explanation of the position of the convener, stressing their impartiality
- A request to confirm the complainant's outstanding issues from Local Resolution (if this has not already been done)
- Information concerning consultation with the independent lay chair
- That they will be taking clinical advice
- The aims behind the Convening Decision
- That the convener cannot award compensation
- That the complaints process must stop if legal action is started
- That an Independent Review Panel cannot recommend disciplinary action
- That the options open to the convener are to refer back to Local Resolution, to refuse a panel or to convene an Independent Review Panel
- The time limits for the Convening Decision (20 working days).

secondary care

2

2

secondary care

Letter informing the complained against of the outstanding issues

This letter advises the complained against that a request for an Independent Review Panel has been received and encloses a copy of the complainant's letter stating the outstanding issues. The Health Service Circular *NHS Complaints Procedures: Confidentiality*, serial number HSC 1998/059, suggests that some conveners have circulated the complainant's statement to other parties and states that should this be done only in exceptional circumstances. It goes on to say that it should be sent only to:

- The person who is subject to the complaint
- Any other person named in the complaint
- The lay chair
- The clinical advisor(s).

Copies will be sent to the panel members and the clinical assessors if a panel is appointed.

Letter to the clinical advisor(s)

This letter is sent to each person who is acting as a clinical advisor to the convener. Some conveners ask the clinical advisors to complete a form so that the procedure is standardised. A copy of the form can then be passed on to the lay chair to ensure that both parties responsible for the Convening Decision receive identical information.

The following information may be included in a letter requesting clinical advice:

- A copy of the outstanding issues from Local Resolution
- A request to concentrate on the outstanding areas, as outlined by the complainant, pertaining to their speciality
- A reminder that their comments are for the convener and the lay chair, both of whom are lay people. Therefore any medical terminology should be explained
- A request to say whether or not the complainant has received a full explanation
- If the complainant has not received a full explanation and additional information is available, a request for any further suggestions for Local Resolution
- A request to say if an apology is required and, if it is, has it been given
- If an error has occurred, a request to say whether satisfactory steps have been put in place to prevent it happening again, and whether the complainant has been fully advised about the action taken by the Trust

- A reminder that, if an Independent Review Panel is refused, the substance of the clinical advice will be passed on to the complainant.

The correspondence and associated paper work from Local Resolution would be appended to the letter, together with the appropriate clinical records.

Letter from the convener to the lay chair

As they work in slightly different ways, it is helpful to the lay chair if the convener sends a letter explaining how they work and what they expect of the lay chair. The type of information that would be included in such a letter would be:

- The name and contact details of the convener
- Whether any Convening Decision forms are to be used
- A request for the lay chair to look at the outstanding issues and make a decision
- Information as to whether the decision could be made on the telephone or if a meeting is required
- The clinical advice received by the convener
- Details of who to contact if any further information is required
- An indication of who is to make the next contact and when.

File notes

The file note usually contains the following information:

- The name of the lay chair and the convener
- The case reference
- The date the decision was made
- Whether it was a telephone conversation or a meeting
- The decision on each outstanding issue
- If there was agreement or disagreement about the outcome
- The date and signature of both parties.

This note would form part of the audit trail and is a record of the Convening Decision. It would be filed in the complaints file.

Letter to the complainant following the Convening Decision

The content of this letter would vary slightly depending on the result of the Convening Decision. It would usually inform the complainant:

- That consultation had taken place with an independent lay chair
- That clinical advice had been taken (if appropriate)

secondary care

secondary care

- Of the Convening Decision for each of the outstanding issues
- Of the complainant's rights following the Convening Decision.

If the complaint had been referred back to Local Resolution, the letter would include details of the:

- Recommendations for further action by the Trust
- Complainant's right to re-request an Independent Review Panel if further Local Resolution is unsuccessful.

If the request for an Independent Review Panel has been refused, the letter would include:

- Information as to where the complaint had been answered
- The substance of the clinical advice
- A paragraph outlining the complainant's right to go to the Ombudsman and full information about how he can be contacted.

If the request for the Independent Review Panel had been agreed, the letter would include the terms of reference for the panel.

Letter from the convener to the parties complained against

Following the Convening Decision, the convener should write to all of the parties complained against advising them of the decision, outlining any further action required (if appropriate) and enclosing a copy of the letter to the complainant.

Letter to the chief executive

Following the Convening Decision, the convener writes to the chief executive of the Trust advising them of the decision, outlining any further action required (if appropriate) and enclosing a copy of the letter to the complainant.

If the decision has been made to convene a panel the letter should also advise the chief executive of:

- The terms of reference of the panel
- The need to appoint a purchaser representative
- Whether or not there is a need to appoint clinical assessors
- The need for administrative support for the panel.

The Independent Review Panel

An Independent Review Panel is made up of three members – the Trust's convener, the lay chair and a representative from the purchaser. If the complaint has a clinical component then the panel will be assisted by a minimum of two clinical assessors who are appointed from outside the Region.

PAPERWORK AND POLICIES

Prior to any Independent Review Panel a basic set of information will be required. Once obtained this paperwork can be used for any subsequent panel that may be established. The paperwork will cover the following areas:

- Indemnity
- Confidentiality
- Expressions of interest

- Return and storage of papers
- Payable expenses
- Letters of appointment
- Secretarial support for the panel
- Tape-recording
- Panel papers, including medical records.

Indemnity

The lay chair, clinical assessors and purchaser representative will all require indemnity. The Trust's insurers should cover Independent Review Panel members but they need to be informed that Independent Review Panels will be taking place and that the panels are a subcommittee of the Trust.

Typical wording in an appointment letter could be as follows:

In the event that a claim does arise from the actions undertaken under this appointment, the Trust will indemnify you in accordance with the Department of Health policy, so long as you have acted in good faith, reasonably and without negligence.

Confidentiality

Health Service Circular HSC 199/053, *For the Record*, discusses the management of records within Trusts. Section 4 of the circular emphasises the importance of maintaining professional ethical standards of confidentiality. The report discusses the confidential duty of people with access to patient information to the patient whose information they hold, and goes on to stress that the duty of confidence is long established in common law.

The Caldicott Review of Patient Identifiable Information, published in December 1997, identified a general lack of awareness of confidentiality and information security throughout the NHS. Whereas the clinical assessors should be aware of the need for confidentiality through their professional training, the Trust will have a duty of care to ensure that the lay chair and the purchaser representative do not disclose confidential information to unauthorised parties and that any paperwork is kept secure and safe at all times and is not accessible to any unauthorised person.

It will be up to each individual Trust to decide the amount of information given to ensure that confidentiality will be upheld. For example:

All activity undertaken under this appointment is confidential and should not be disclosed to any third parties. There may be circumstances when you are approached directly for information or comment about the panel's activities. All such approaches should be referred immediately to the Trust's ... manager.

Or:

Confidentiality:

1. The contents of the Independent Review Panel papers must not be discussed with anyone who is not directly involved in the Independent Review Panel process.
2. The papers should be kept in a safe and secure place and should be inaccessible by unauthorised persons at all times.
3. All papers should be returned to the Trust's ... manager on completion of the Independent Review Panel report for safe storage.
4. The identity of the complainant must not be revealed to any person who is not directly involved in the Independent Review Panel process.

Expressions of interest

Before any papers are sent out to the panel members and the assessors, a check should be made to ensure that they do not know the parties involved in the complaint. This check can take the form of a telephone conversation. Problems may arise with clinical assessors, particularly if one of the staff involved in the complaint is well known in their field. The informal test tends to be whether they would see the person socially, or invite them to their house.

The Trust needs a method of working to make sure that these checks do take place and to clearly identify both the person doing the checks and the person sending out the papers. If this was not the same person then the responsibility for checking would usually rest with the person sending out the papers.

Return and storage of papers

As the Department of Health has indicated that complaints papers should be stored for the same length of time as medical records, a system needs to be in place outlining how and when the papers are returned and who is responsible for checking that this has been done.

Some lay chairs may want to keep their papers in case the complaint is referred to the Ombudsman. Perhaps the simplest way of handling this is to suggest that they place their personal notes in a sealed envelope and put their name and the complaint reference on the outside. This can then be filed with the complaints papers and returned if required. Any duplicate papers can be destroyed and this should be done by the Trust staff. It is not acceptable to allow the panel members or assessors to destroy their own papers as the Trust will have no means of knowing that this has been done correctly.

Payable expenses

It is up to each individual Trust to decide the rate at which expenses are reimbursed. Guidance was issued by the Head of Employment Issues at the

secondary care

2

NHS Executive Headquarters in September 1996 and the payment to panel members and clinical assessors was covered in EL(96)19. Panel chairs are eligible for travel expenses, subsistence allowance and loss of earnings. Conveners who are non-executive directors cannot receive any additional payment but it is up to Trusts to make their own arrangements when appointing additional conveners.

Clinical assessors can claim an honorarium of £150 per day (consultant medical and dental staff can claim £175), along with travel and subsistence allowance.

It is helpful to the panel members and assessors if, on appointment, information is sent from the Trust outlining:

- The rate travel allowance is paid
- Whether additional expenditure can be claimed (telephone, postage)
- What is acceptable as loss of earnings and what documentation will be required, perhaps with a maximum daily rate payable
- The payment rate for clinical assessors
- Whether overnight accommodation will be provided.

In addition, a travel and subsistence claim form should be provided, with details of when and to whom it should be returned.

Letters of appointment

These can take the form of a standard letter and should be sent out immediately after the appointments have been agreed and it has been confirmed that the parties do not have an interest in the case. The letter would contain some or all of the following information:

- The name of the complainant
- The subject of the complaint
- Confirmation of the appointment
- An indication that the Independent Review Panel is a subcommittee of the Trust
- Indemnity information
- Confidentiality information
- Details of reimbursement of travel, subsistence, postage, fee (for clinical assessors), amount paid for loss of earnings (lay chairs, if appropriate)
- A request to confirm that they do not have an interest
- A statement that they agree to the conditions outlined in the letter
- A request to date and sign, one copy and return it to the Trust, retaining the other copy for their records
- A copy of the Briefing Pack for Clinical Assessors produced by the Institute of Health and Care Development and published by the NHS Executive (for clinical assessors).

Secretarial support for the panel

If the Trust's complaints manager has been dealing with the complaint under Local Resolution it is advisable for another person to provide the secretarial and administrative support for the panel. This distances the Independent Review Panel from the Local Resolution process. In some larger Trusts with more than one complaints manager, one will deal with Local Resolution and the other with the Independent Review Panel. Smaller Trusts need to identify someone to support the panel at the beginning of the process. The person selected will need to have the time to administer all correspondence and to minute any panel meetings, bearing in mind the time scales laid down for the completion of each stage of the process.

Minutes should be taken at all meetings of the panel so that an audit trail can take place. These minutes will be required if the complaint is subsequently referred to the Ombudsman and investigated.

Tape-recording

Whether to tape-record the Independent Review Panel's work is a decision for each individual Trust. Before reaching a decision, the following points should be considered:

- Why is tape-recording required?
- Will the tape be transcribed?
- If yes, will the person transcribing be able to recognise who is speaking?
- If no, is it merely a back-up to the minute taker?
- Will the parties be informed in advance about the tape-recording?
- What will happen if someone refuses to be recorded?
- What will happen if the machine jams?
- What will happen to the tape after the Independent Review Panel?
- What is the Trust's position if they are asked for a copy of the tape?

If the decision is made to tape-record proceedings then it is advisable to inform the parties well in advance that this will be happening. The Trust should ask their permission, advise them of the purpose of the tape-recording and tell them what will happen to the tape at the end of the Independent Review Panel process.

Panel papers

The panel members and the clinical assessors will require the following papers prior to the Independent Review Panel:

- The terms of reference
- Copies of any correspondence concerning the complaint
- Minutes of any Local Resolution meetings

- Medical records relevant to the complaint
- Nursing records relevant to the complaint.

The correspondence and minutes of any meetings should be numbered and in date order as this aids discussion at any subsequent meetings. A cover sheet listing the correspondence is useful as it makes it much easier to find a particular piece of correspondence when required.

The papers need to be sent out as soon as possible after the request for an Independent Review Panel has been granted. Included with the papers should be:

- Dates and times of any subsequent meetings
- Details of the venue
- A map of the venue
- Information concerning contact names and telephone numbers.

Care should be taken to ensure that the papers will arrive securely. Boxes or Jiffy bags are preferable to standard envelopes, which often become damaged in transit.

It is advisable to mark the packaging in such a way as to indicate that the contents are confidential and to be opened by the addressee only.

THE LAY CHAIR

Once the Convening Decision has been made to convene a panel, and the terms of reference have been written, the responsibility moves from the convener to the lay chair. The Trust is required to provide administrative support for the lay chair. The role of the lay chair is to:

- Chair any meetings of the panel
- Decide, in conjunction with the panel members, how the panel should operate
- Decide the procedure to be adopted by the panel
- Question those interviewed, as appropriate
- Lead the panel in writing its report.
- Ensure there are no suggestions or recommendations about disciplinary action in the report
- Agree the draft circulation of the report with the panel members
- Aim to meet the target time scales for the Independent Review Panel
- Decide if, in the interest of the patient, part of the report should be withheld
- Sign and distribute the final report.

THE PURCHASER REPRESENTATIVE

The Health Authority purchasing the care received by the patient appoints the purchaser representative. Care should be taken to ensure that the correct Health Authority is contacted by carefully checking the postcode of the patient (which may be different from that of the complainant). The role of the purchaser representative is to:

- Read the papers
- Participate in any meetings of the panel
- Decide, with the lay chair, how the panel should do its work
- Question those interviewed, as appropriate
- Contribute to the panel's report
- Agree, with the lay chair, the distribution of the draft report
- Check the final panel report.

THE CONVENER

The role of the convener is similar to that of the purchaser representative, i.e. to:

- Read the papers
- Participate in any meetings of the panel
- Decide, with the lay chair, how the panel should do its work
- Question those interviewed, as appropriate
- Contribute to the panel's report
- Agree, with the lay chair, the distribution of the draft report
- Check the final panel report.

In addition, the convener is in a position to check that any recommendations made by the panel, and agreed by the Trust, are implemented.

CLINICAL ASSESSORS

The clinical assessors are appointed from outside the region. They are selected from the list provided by the Regional Office and are appointed for their expertise. In clinical complaints there must be at least two clinical assessors. If a complaint concerns only one profession then two assessors from that profession would be appointed. If the complaint concerns more than one profession then an assessor from each speciality would be required.
    The role of the clinical assessors is to:

- Advise the panel on the clinical aspects of the terms of reference
- Produce draft reports prior to the panel hearing
- Participate in any meetings of the panel
- Question those interviewed, as appropriate
- Contribute to the panel's report
- Check the panel's final report
- Produce either an individual or joint clinical assessor's report(s) using lay terminology.

A suggested content of the final assessor's report would be:

- A summary of the clinical aspects of the case
- The findings and recommendations for each term of reference.

The clinical assessors cannot suggest disciplinary action.

SUGGESTED PROCEDURE FOR THE INDEPENDENT REVIEW PANEL PROCESS

There is no fixed procedure for the Independent Review Panel process. This allows flexibility and enables the panel to accommodate the needs of individual complainants but, unfortunately, has also given rise to problems, as certain criteria must be upheld. For example:

- The complainant and the complained against must be treated equally
- Clinical assessors must be present when clinical issues are discussed
- The participants must be allowed to put their case orally or, if they wish, in writing
- The complainant can be accompanied by a relative or friend, plus an advisor, when interviewed
- Any person complained against can be accompanied by an advisor when interviewed
- All interviews must be in private
- Notes of any interview should be kept.

Therefore, although there is flexibility in the system the majority of panels adopt the following procedure:

- A meeting of panel members as soon as it is known that a panel is to be convened
- An initial meeting of the panel and clinical assessors immediately prior to the Independent Review Panel
- The Independent Review Panel
- A meeting immediately after the Independent Review Panel.

A meeting of panel members as soon as it is known that a panel is to be convened

This meeting involves the panel members only and allows them to meet each other. As with all meetings of the panel, a record should be kept of the discussions. At this meeting the following information can be decided:

- Which staff members will be interviewed
- Whether written statements can be taken from staff members
- Whether any additional papers are required
- The order in which the interviews will take place

- The length of time allocated to each interview
- The venue for the Independent Review Panel
- The date for the Independent Review Panel
- If any exceptional circumstances need to be taken into account.

Experience shows that it usually takes between 1 and 2 hours for the complainant to give information to the panel and between 15 minutes and 1 hour for staff members. The length of time required will depend on the complexity of the case.

Who can attend

A relative or friend, plus a person to act as an advisor, can accompany the complainant. If more than one family member is involved in the complaint they usually attend the Independent Review Panel together. The person accompanying may speak to the panel with the lay chair's consent but, if they are legally qualified, they may not act as an advocate. It should be remembered that the aim of the panel is to establish what happened and therefore first-hand accounts will always carry more weight than second-hand accounts.

Staff members may also be accompanied by an advisor. It is usual to see the staff members individually.

It is usual for the complainant to be interviewed first and then the staff. This is much less confrontational than having both parties in the room together and appears to allow a much more open dialogue between the panel and the person being interviewed. It is possible that the complainant will want to hear what the staff are saying to the panel, but there are facilities for this to happen under Local Resolution and they will be sent a summary of the information given to the panel in the final report.

Accommodation required for the panel

The venue for the Independent Review Panel is often in a non-clinical area of the Trust. Most people involved in the process agree that it should not be in a patient area. Holding the Independent Review Panel on Trust premises enables staff to attend with the minimum disruption to the hospital routine.

Ideally, the room should be large enough to seat the panel members, clinical assessors, secretarial support, the complainant and their relatives, friends and advisor. It is much easier if everyone can sit round the same table. This allows people to place any papers on the table and enables the panel members and the parties being interviewed to take notes if they wish. It has been argued that the use of low chairs and coffee tables is a better arrangement but this can give an appearance of informality and the impression that the panel is not taking the complaint seriously.

The use of separate waiting areas where the parties can speak to their advisor prior to the review is often appreciated, as is the provision of beverages and name plates for the panel members and assessors.

The list provided in Chapter 3 (pp. 18–20) with suggestions for access for disabled people could be used to check the suitability of the chosen venue and the information on the use of interpreters in the same chapter (pp. 17–18) should also be noted.

Exceptional circumstances

There may be occasions when it is not appropriate for the complainant to appear before the full panel. An example would be if the patient was bedridden, very elderly or had learning difficulties and it was thought that a panel would be intimidating. In these circumstances it would be possible for one of the panel members to interview the complainant on their own. If the complaint had a clinical nature the panel member would have to be accompanied by one of the clinical assessors. Minutes of the meeting would be taken and the information fed back to the other panel members.

If one of the panel members was unable to attend on the day, perhaps because of illness or another unavoidable situation, the panel should go ahead, rather than being cancelled and reconvened. If the lay chair was unable to attend it would be more acceptable for the purchaser representative to chair the panel than the convener, as they would be seen to be more independent. If one of the clinical assessors was unable to attend the panel could still go ahead, although this should be the exception rather than normal procedure.

Performance targets

The performance targets are laid down in the Guidance documentation and are as follows:

- Appointment of panel members – 20 working days after the Convening Decision
- Draft report of the panel – 50 working days after the panel has been set up
- Final panel report – A further 10 working days
- Response by the Trust – A further 20 working days.

The performance targets are for guidance only. If they are not going to be met then all the parties should be informed that there will be a delay and given the reasons for the delay. The lay chair is responsible for maintaining time scales although, in reality, the monitoring is usually done by the Trust staff.

An initial meeting of the panel and clinical assessors immediately prior to the Independent Review Panel

This meeting usually takes place in the hour immediately prior to the Independent Review Panel. The clinical assessors usually produce a draft report based on the written documentation and clinical records. At this meeting the draft assessor's reports are discussed and the order of questioning is agreed. It is usual for the clinical assessors to concentrate on the clinical aspect of the complaint and at this meeting will decide if they will answer questions posed to them by the complainant and if they will explain certain areas of the case to the complainant. Both the answering of questions and the provision of explanations will often help the complainant understand what has happened. The fact that the explanation comes from someone outside the Trust often makes it more acceptable than if the same explanation is given by the Trust staff. In addition, as minutes are taken during the interview, there will be a record of the answers and explanations, which will allow the complainant to re-read the information at a later date.

It is usual for the lay chair to sit in the centre of the panel with a panel member and clinical assessor on either side.

The Independent Review Panel

As has already been said, the running of the panel is not prescribed but the most common approach is to interview the complainant first followed by the complained against and any other members of the staff the panel need to see. By far the most usual procedure is as follows:

- The lay chair meets the person to be interviewed outside the room
- The lay chair brings the person into the room and introduces them to the panel members and the assessors
- The lay chair explains the procedure
- The lay chair reads out the terms of reference for the panel
- The lay chair invites the person being interviewed to outline any information they wish to tell the panel
- The clinical assessors ask questions
- The panel members ask questions
- The lay chair explains the next stage in the procedure and thanks the person for attending.

Greeting the interviewee

The lay chair usually goes to meet the person being interviewed. This gives them a brief opportunity to meet all the people involved. Introductions can be made and the lay chair can mention their independence from the Trust. The lay chair then brings the participants into the room and introduces the panel members and clinical assessors, indicating who they are, where they are from and their role on the panel.

The procedure

After sitting down, the lay chair explains how the panel will operate, explaining that the panel wishes to hear the complainant's account of what happened and that then they will be interviewing the staff involved. The person minuting the panel is introduced and the interviewee is informed that they will have an opportunity to see the minutes of the information they give to the panel for approval before the report is published.

The terms of reference

Reading out the terms of reference reminds the person being interviewed and the panel members of the parameters of the panel. This hopefully allows the panel to concentrate on the areas of importance and prevents extra issues, or those that have been answered under Local Resolution, being introduced at this stage of the proceedings.

The opening statement

Asking the interviewee to give their account of what happened allows them to tell their story. It is helpful if the person can be allowed to speak without interruption, as they will then feel that they have had the opportunity to say what they want to say. Many people see the Independent Review Panel as their 'day in court' and have often rehearsed what they want to say. In cases of bereavement this can often be a very emotional time for them and it is a good idea to have water and paper tissues available. In some cases, the telling of the story is a form of release and can help a bereaved person through that stage of the bereavement process.

The questions

After the opening statement, the panel members and clinical assessors have an opportunity to question the interviewee. The panel members should bear in mind that part of the panel report is the findings of fact about the terms of reference. Closed questions are often a useful way of clarifying the facts of the complaint. For example:

- Did the doctor examine you?
- Did you ask to speak to the doctor?
- Which nurse did you speak to?
- Which day did you visit?
- What time did you telephone?

This is also an opportunity for the clinical assessors to answer questions from the interviewee and to explain areas of concern that the interviewee may have.

The closing remarks

The lay chair thanks the interviewee(s) for attending and explains the next stages. The lay chair may:

- Outline the time scales
- Tell the complainant that they will see the minutes of the interview
- Remind them that the report is confidential
- Inform them of their right to go to the Ombudsman
- Offer condolences if a bereavement has occurred.

The whole procedure is then repeated for each person being interviewed.

A meeting immediately after the Independent Review Panel

Although in complex complaints the panel can be very tired by this point in the proceedings it is very useful and effective to have a meeting with the panel members and the clinical assessors to discuss:

- The findings of fact
- The opinions of the panel
- Recommendations.

The findings of fact

The findings of fact are numbered and written in date order. They provide a summary of the case pertaining to the terms of reference. Events can be listed as facts when both parties agree or when the facts are supported by contemporaneous written evidence or by an independent person. Clinicians are used to summarising information and can be invaluable in this stage of the process. For example:

1. 1 August, Mrs Jones was admitted to Ward A of the Royal Hospital at 9.00 a.m.
2. Mrs Jones was examined by the senior house officer at 1.00 p.m.
3. The medical records record that Mrs Jones' blood pressure was raised, that her abdomen was tender and that she was referred for an abdominal X-ray.
4. 2 August, Mrs Jones' abdomen was radiographed at 3.00 p.m.
5. 3 August, the senior house officer noted that the X-ray report indicated that Mrs Jones had an abdominal obstruction and she consented to an operation.

secondary care

2

6. Mrs Jones was examined by the anaesthetist at 10.30 a.m. and was taken to theatre at 2.00 p.m. for an operation to remove the obstruction.

7. Regrettably Mrs Jones had a heart attack during the operation and, in spite of attempts by the surgeon to resuscitate her, she died on the operating table.

The opinions of the panel

The panel members and the assessors then take each term of reference in turn and discuss it, based on the findings of fact. For example:
To investigate the events leading up to Mrs Jones' death from her admittance in hospital on 1 August.

- The panel was advised by the clinical assessors that Mrs Jones was seen and examined on 1 August and that appropriate tests were requested. The X-ray results confirmed that there was an obstruction and an operation was scheduled for 3 August.
- The panel was also advised that there was nothing in the medical records to indicate that Mrs Jones had a heart problem and that the heart attack was unexpected. They noted that Mrs Jones had also been seen by an anaesthetist on the morning of the operation and that the surgeon had tried to resuscitate Mrs Jones.
- The clinical assessors were of the opinion that there was a delay in obtaining the X-ray report, which in turn delayed the subsequent operation, but they advised the panel that this would not have affected the outcome.

The recommendations

When making its recommendations, the panel must remember that it is a subcommittee of the Trust and that it should not suggest any disciplinary action. Recommendations should therefore suggest ways in which the Trust could improve the efficiency or effectiveness of the services it offers. In addition, the panel could make recommendations as to ways in which the Trust could satisfy the complainant. For example, following on from the above examples the panel could recommend that:

The Trust evaluates the reporting of urgent X-ray requests to ensure that any findings on a radiograph are communicated to the ward on the same day.

THE CLINICAL ASSESSOR'S REPORT

The clinical assessors can either produce individual reports or a joint report. Some Trusts offer facilities for the assessors to dictate their final reports on the day but the practicality of this will depend on the complexity of the

Independent Review Panel. Separate reports are seen as being more independent by the complainant but care should be taken to make sure that any contradictory sections are clearly explained and to indicate why there is a difference of opinion.

Although joint reports can expose the clinicians to the accusation of collusion, they can be helpful in very complex complaints by clarifying, in a logical manner, the clinical aspects of the case.

THE INDEPENDENT REVIEW PANEL REPORT

The confidential report is produced by the panel. There are certain compulsory elements to the report, which are outlined in the underpinning legislation and include:

* The findings of fact relevant to the complaint
* The opinion of the panel on the findings of fact
* The reasons for the panel's opinion
* The report of the assessors
* If the panel disagrees with any aspect of the assessor's report, the reason for the disagreement.

Comments from the Ombudsman in his annual reports have indicated further information to be included in the final report. Summaries of papers received by the panel members and a summary of evidence given to the panel makes the report into a document that can be read and understood in its own right. The suggested format of the report is given in Figure 19.1.

The draft report

There has been much discussion as to whether the draft report should be sent to the parties involved. Issuing a draft report gives people the opportunity to correct any errors before the final report is published. The problems associated with issuing a full draft report are related to how the panel deals with any corrections:

* What would the panel do if the complainant wished to change someone else's statement?
* How would the panel react if it disagreed with the 'correction'?
* What would the panel do if one person wanted a finding of fact changed but another agreed with the original version?

It could be argued that if the panel is not going to act on the changes identified then it is not appropriate to send out the full draft report. In addition, there will be will be two reports in circulation – the draft report and the final report. It would therefore be sensible to mark the draft report clearly, so that there can be no confusion at a later date.

2

secondary care

CONFIDENTIAL

Name of Trust
Report of the Independent Review Panel
held on (date)

Complaint brought by............

Panel Members
> Name   Position

Clinical Assessors
> Name   Position

Terms of Reference
> List

Panel Procedure
> A brief summary of the steps the panel took to investigate the complaint, including any meetings held and a list of documentation reviewed by the panel.

Précis of Interviews/Written Statements
> Covering only the information relevant to the terms of reference.

*Findings of Fact
> Numbered and in date order.

*Opinions of the panel on the Findings of Fact
> Take each of the terms of reference and comment, based on the findings of fact and giving reasons for any observations. If a finding of fact cannot be found, give the reasons.

If the panel disagrees with any matter included in the assessor's report
> Give reasons for the disagreements.

Recommendations
> The panel recommends to the Trust (if appropriate).

Signature
> Of lay chair (and other panel members if desired).

Date

Appendices

* Clinical Assessor's Report(s)
> Signed and dated

> > > *** Mandatory as per the directions**

Fig. 19.1

A compromise has been found to work very well. The person who was interviewed receives a copy of the full minutes of their interview for checking. Any corrections are accepted by the panel. The corrected report is then summarised to exclude the introduction of any new areas that are outside the terms of reference and the summarised version is included in the final report.

ISSUES ARISING DURING THE INDEPENDENT REVIEW PANEL PROCESS

As has been stated earlier, the purpose of the complaints process is to provide a full explanation to the complainant; it is not to lay blame or to suggest disciplinary action. The panel and assessors must remain impartial and both parties must be treated equally and fairly. It has to be remembered that, to request an Independent Review Panel, the complainant must state what issues remain outstanding and why they remain dissatisfied; the terms of reference for the panel are drawn from these outstanding issues. Therefore, originally it is the complainant who determines which issues form the basis of the panel's deliberations.

Several problem areas have arisen during and after Independent Review Panels:

- The introduction of new issues by the complainant
- The introduction of areas of concern by the clinical assessors
- The naming of parties in the body of the report.

The introduction of new issues by the complainant

The directions are very clear in stating that any new issues should be referred back to Local Resolution. However, once the panel procedure is in process this is very difficult to do. A practical way of handling this is for the lay chair to allow any queries to be answered, if appropriate – usually by one of the clinical assessors. As this discussion is recorded in the minutes, the complainant would have a written copy of the explanation given. The account included in the final report would cover only the areas included in the terms of reference for the panel and not this new area.

The introduction of areas of concern by the clinical assessors

One of the problems in handling complaints is that the complainant sometimes complains about the wrong person or the wrong area. As the purpose of the panel is to answer the complaint, how should any areas of concern be handled? The answer will depend on the severity of the concern. It should be remembered that it is very easy to find areas for improvement when reviewing someone else's work, as it is impossible for anyone to provide a 'gold standard' service 100% of the time. The clinical assessors should advise the panel if their concerns are such that further action needs to be taken, bearing in mind that they have a duty of care to report any serious areas of concern. What must be remembered is that if the areas of concern fall outside the terms of reference for the panel, then the panel report is not the place to raise them. They should instead be raised with either the chief executive or the medical director of the Trust concerned.

The naming of parties in the body of the report

The question then arises as to whether or not the parties should be named in the body of the report. The *Guidance on Implementing the NHS Complaints Procedure* advises that when anonymised information would suffice, any identifiable information should be omitted. The Ombudsman names the complainant and the Trust in his reports but not the individuals interviewed, referring to them only by their job title.

It has been argued, usually by lay chairs, that the parties should be named, as the process should be open and transparent. However, before naming individuals in a report the following questions should be asked:

- Is it fair for a member of staff to be named if they are correctly following a Trust policy but that the policy or procedure is incorrect?
- Does it add to the provision of a full explanation to the patient if the staff are named?
- Will it improve the service to other patients if staff are named?
- Could the naming of staff imply disciplinary action?
- Would the staff be treated equitably if they are named in the report?
- What would the Trust's position be if the staff are named and the report is published in the press?

THE CIRCULATION OF THE FINAL REPORT

The final report is sent out by the lay chair. It is helpful if the letter can indicate that the report is confidential. Once the report has been circulated, the lay chair should have no further contact with the parties involved. Copies of the final report are sent to:

- The complainant
- Any person complained against
- Any person interviewed
- The patient, if they are not the complainant
- The assessors
- The chair and chief executive of the Trust

- The chair and chief executive of the purchasing Health Authority
- The Regional Office of the NHS Executive.

It is possible for the lay chair to withhold parts of the report in the interest of protecting the confidentiality of the patient and any third party or of protecting the health of the complainant or a patient who is not the complainant.

Any written statements provided to the panel should not be disclosed unless the person providing the information has consented to the disclosure. The guidance clearly states that, when anonymised information about patients or third parties would suffice, then identifiable information should be omitted.

HSC1998/059, which was issued to lay chairs, indicates that the full report should be seen only by a limited number of people. It quotes the example of people who are interviewed by the panel but not directly involved in the complaint. These people should see only the parts of the report that relate to the information they gave, and not the full report. If the lay chair decides to withhold part of the report then it would be sensible to record the reasons for this decision.

ACTION FOLLOWING THE DISSEMINATION OF THE FINAL REPORT

Within 20 working days of the receipt of the report the Trust chief executive should write to the complainant saying what action the Trust proposes to take on the panel's recommendations. If the Trust decides not to take any action on the recommendations then the reasons for this decision must be given. In addition, the complainant should be informed that they have the right to contact the Ombudsman if they remain dissatisfied. Full contact details should be included in the letter.

20

Clinical participation

WHO SHOULD PARTICIPATE?

In the context of the complaints system, the term 'clinician' is used to denote any health care professional who may have been involved with the care of the patient. When handling complaints, the stage of the complaints process will determine whether the original clinician, their line manager, a more senior member of staff or a clinician from another Trust is required. The underlying principle is that the person selected should be of the same profession and the same speciality as the person complained about. Therefore, for example, when involving a medical consultant it would be inappropriate to use a neurologist for an obstetric complaint and vice versa.

When dealing with complainants, clinicians should remember that they are usually dealing with lay people and should therefore take care to avoid the use of medical jargon if at all possible. If jargon is unavoidable, an attempt should be made to explain the terms used. Unfortunately, with the number of medical programmes in the media (both fact and fiction), the information available on the internet, the ability for patients to access their medical records and the volumes of written material available, the general public tend to use medical terms when they only partially understand the meaning of them. This can give the impression that they have a much greater understanding than they actually have. For example, to a lay person the term 'distress' can mean that someone is tearful or upset; to a clinician it is often used as a shorthand for respiratory distress, meaning difficulty in breathing.

Dealing correctly with complainants is time consuming but clinicians should remember that time taken early on in the complaints process can

secondary care

2

often save many hours of time later on by reducing the likelihood of the complaint moving on to the next stage.

THE CLINICIAN'S ROLE IN LOCAL RESOLUTION
Preventing complaints

All health care professionals should be aware of potential scenarios that may lead to a complaint, and should take steps to intervene if they think such a scenario is developing. The following list gives examples, but is by no means exhaustive:

- A clinic is running late – the clinician goes into the waiting area, apologises for the delay and gives some indication of the time people will have to wait
- A piece of X-ray equipment breaks down, as a result patients will have to come back on another occasion – the radiographer apologises and explains the reasons for the cancellation
- A nurse informs relatives the patient's condition is improving, that night the patient's condition deteriorates rapidly and the relatives have to be sent for – the nurse approaches the relatives when they arrive on the ward, apologises and explains that they were acting in good faith and the change in the patient's condition was unexpected
- Relatives are demanding to see a senior member of staff and appear to have a number of 'trivial' questions – if possible, arrange a private meeting. Consider having a nurse present who can check understanding and follow-up with the relatives. Remember, their behaviour may be masking worries and concerns about the patient.

Oral complaints

Oral complaints should, if at all possible, be dealt with immediately. If a clinician is asked to see either a patient or relative about a complaint then the sooner this happens, the more likely they are to be able to resolve the complaint. It will be possible to answer the majority of oral complaints by explaining why a particular course of action has taken place and to answer questions fully and completely. Try to ensure that all questions have been answered and offer apologies if appropriate. Make sure that a record of the conversation is made, including the date, time, who was present and the substance of the information given.

Responding to written complaints

In order to respond fully to written complaints, the clinician will require the appropriate medical and/or nursing records and will need

2

to talk to the staff who were dealing with the patient. To provide a satisfactory response it is important that the following questions are answered:

- Is the response factually correct?
- Has any medical jargon been explained?
- Has a full explanation been given?
- If an error has occurred, has an apology been given?
- If an error has occurred, is there an explanation of the steps that will be taken to try to prevent it happening again?
- Have all the points in the letter been answered?

Experience has shown that complaints that progress to Independent Review Panels have done so because one (or more) of the above questions has not been addressed. In order to save time, clinicians have said what they thought would have happened rather than what actually did happen, forgetting that, although to them the patient was one patient in a busy clinic, to the patient it may well have been a unique experience. At Independent Review Panels it is not unusual to interview junior staff and find that they became aware of the complaint only when it was decided to hold a panel, and that they had not been involved in any aspect of Local Resolution.

The response to a written complaint needs to be given in such a way that the complainant can fully understand the contents of the letter. Abbreviations should therefore be avoided wherever possible and medical terminology and test results will require explanation.

A full explanation may well have to include information about why a certain procedure was not done or was not appropriate. If something has gone wrong, patients are entitled to an apology and the Medical Protection Society and the Medical Defence Union now encourage staff to apologise in such situations. From the complainant's perspective, many people 'do not wish it to happen to anyone else', and it is therefore important to explain if, and how, systems or procedures are being changed. Equally, if it is perceived by the complainant that an error has been made, but that this was unavoidable, then again a full explanation is required as to why it was unavoidable. For example, a patient is diagnosed as having cancer after they had been in hospital for several weeks, an earlier diagnosis was not possible because all the tests were negative.

Finally, it is also important to double-check that all the points raised in the initial letter have been answered. One approach is to use each complaint as a heading and then answer the complaint under the appropriate heading. This not only makes it easier to check that all the complaints have been covered but tends to make the responses easier to understand, as they become more focused.

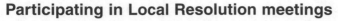

secondary care

2

Participating in Local Resolution meetings

A meeting with the complainant gives an opportunity to give a verbal explanation and to answer as many underlying questions as possible. Although the emphasis is on informality, it is advisable to have notes made of any meeting and to send a copy to the complainant for checking.

It is important to minimise the number of staff present at these meetings, as a complainant can easily feel intimidated and the Trust staff could well be accused of 'ganging up' against the complainant. If a number of staff are involved in a complaint the easiest way of handling the meeting is to arrange the order in which they are seen. When the first person leaves the room they telephone the next person on the list, who then comes in. This process has the advantage of giving the complainant an opportunity to gather their thoughts between seeing people and, in addition, is a more efficient use of staff time.

Preparation prior to the meeting

It is important that the medical or nursing records are available and that the clinician is familiar with the complaint and has spoken directly to the staff involved prior to the meeting. It is important to be as factually accurate as possible and to check whether or not the staff recall either the patient or the incident that led up to the complaint.

At the meeting

Try to be honest – if you or your staff do not remember an incident then say so. It is then possible to go on to say what would usually happen in certain circumstances. Be prepared to apologise if there were faults or omissions in the service that the patient received. It is important that jargon and abbreviations are not used and it can be helpful if there is a lay member of staff present (for example, the complaints manager) who can summarise at regular intervals and try to put any medical terminology into lay terms.

Allow the complainant to ask questions and listen carefully to the question being asked, it is better to ask for clarification before an answer is given than to answer the wrong question! Watch the complainant to assess whether or not they have understood an explanation. It may be necessary to reword a response if you think that the complainant has failed to understand the reply. In more complex medical situations it is sometimes helpful to use diagrams or anatomical models to aid understanding.

Before leaving the meeting, check that the complainant has no further questions and, if there has been a bereavement, offer condolences.

After the meeting

Carefully check the file note to make sure that it is factually accurate and ensure that a copy is sent to the complainant with a request that the Trust be informed if there are any inaccuracies.

INDEPENDENT CLINICAL ADVICE FOR LAY CONCILIATORS

Although conciliation is used extensively in primary care, it is rarely used in Trusts. However, a lay conciliator may become involved if the complainant is not prepared to meet any of the staff in the Trust handling the complaint and therefore, in this context, the independent clinician who advises the lay conciliator would normally work for a neighbouring Trust. Lay conciliators also tend to become involved with the more complex clinical complaints, which often involve bereavement and the emotions associated with bereavement.

Although lay conciliators have different working methods, it is usual for the clinician to have a copy of the medical records and to prepare a brief report, which may or may not be passed on to the complainant. When preparing such a report it is important to remember that it will be read by lay people and to try to avoid the use of unexplained medical terminology and abbreviations. Remember that the purpose of the complaints procedure is to give an explanation of events, not to apportion blame, and therefore the report should concentrate on why a particular course of action was taken.

A meeting may be arranged with the complainant, the lay conciliator and the external clinician. It is important that the original medical records are available and that the meeting is kept as informal as possible. Although the lay conciliator may ask questions on behalf of the complainant it is more usual for the complainant to ask their own questions. The purpose of the meeting is to ensure that the complainant understands what happened and why a particular course of action was taken. In addition, they may be feeling guilty for taking a particular course of action and may require reassurance that they acted appropriately under the circumstances.

It is usual for the lay conciliator to summarise at regular intervals, often putting words into lay terms. The lay conciliator may also ask for the meaning of medical terms to ensure the complainant fully understands the explanation.

As with the other Local Resolution meetings, it is important to check that the complainant has no further questions and that the summary of the meeting is carefully checked to make sure that it is factually accurate.

secondary care

GIVING CLINICAL ADVICE AT THE CONVENING STAGE

If a request for an Independent Review Panel is made and all or part of the complaint is about clinical care, clinical advice must be taken. The advice is taken by the convener and is passed on to the lay chair before the Convening Decision is made. Clinical advice is needed because both the convener and the lay chair are lay people and therefore will be unfamiliar with medical terminology, the lay-out and contents of medical records and why a particular course of action has (or has not) been taken.

It is possible for clinical advice to be given from staff within the Trust but it is important that an appropriate person is selected from the correct speciality. For example, if it is a nursing complaint the nursing director could be used; if it is a cardiology complaint the medical director could be used or they could give the convener the name of the most appropriate consultant to give advice. It is important that the person giving clinical advice has not been involved in any aspect of the complaint during Local Resolution, if this is the case then a clinical advisor should be obtained from the Regional Office.

In more complex complaints the convenor may need to take advice from more than one clinician, for example, a nurse, a speech therapist and a physiotherapist.

Documentation

The clinical advisor will require:

- A list of the clinical issues that the complainant feels are outstanding from Local Resolution
- Copies of any correspondence between the complainant and the Trust
- The notes of any meetings that have taken place during Local Resolution
- The appropriate, original medical/nursing records.

Reviewing the records

It is not the function of the clinical advisor to comment on the appropriateness of the clinical action but to evaluate whether or not the aims of the complaints process have been met for each of the outstanding issues. Therefore, for each of the outstanding clinical issues identified by the complainant, the clinical advisor should assess whether or not:

- A full explanation has been given in a form that the complainant understands
- An apology has been given, if appropriate
- If something has gone wrong, has an explanation been given about the steps to be taken to try to prevent a re-occurrence

- Any outstanding clinical issues, as identified by the complainant, have not been answered
- Any disputed clinical issues have been identified.

It is helpful to both the convener and the lay chair if comments under each of the above headings can be written down, along with any suggestions for any further action that could be taken under Local Resolution.

For example, if a particular treatment had been given and the complainant had said that they felt that an alternative treatment should have been offered but the correspondence only explained why the treatment was given, a recommendation could be made that a letter was written, or a meeting held, to explain why the alternative treatment was not appropriate.

If, on the other hand, the advisor felt that the complainant was correct and that the explanation given was not in line with modern practice they could recommend that the clinician concerned reassessed the treatment given and apologised to the complainant for not offering the alternative treatment.

Clinical advice is given in writing to make sure that both the lay chair and the convener receive the same clinical advice. In addition, the advice can be placed on file and will therefore form part of the audit trail if the complaints procedure is evaluated. If the convener refuses the request for the Independent Review, the substance of the clinical advice is passed on to the complainant and, again, it is helpful if reasons for the decisions are given. For example, where a particular point has been answered or that the treatment given was in line with current practice. In addition, the comments should be written in lay terms and any medical terminology or abbreviations should be explained.

When offering clinical advice you may come across examples of clinical practice that give you cause for concern. As a clinician, you have a duty of care to raise your concerns with the appropriate person but if this is not an area that has been complained about then this should be done outside the complaints procedure. Clinicians need to remember that, when giving clinical advice, they are looking at only the outstanding issues identified by the complainant, it is therefore not necessary to review the whole of the treatment.

CLINICAL ASSESSMENT FOR THE INDEPENDENT REVIEW PANEL

The Department of Health has compiled a list of people who are willing to act as clinical assessors and this list is consulted when a request is made by a Trust for clinical assessors to advise the lay Independent Review Panel members. Clinical assessors are appointed from outside the Trust's region and there are a minimum of two assessors for an Independent Review Panel with a clinical element.

When appointed, the clinical assessors should receive the following information.

- Details of the parties involved in the complaint. The assessors should make sure that they do not know either of the parties before agreeing to accept the appointment
- A letter of appointment, which should include indemnity cover for the assessor whilst they are working on the complaint
- A claim form for the fees
- The terms of reference for the Independent Review Panel. These will limit the workings of the panel and indicate the areas that the assessors should concentrate on when writing their reports and questioning the parties
- Copies of the correspondence between the complainant and the Trust, including the file notes of any meetings that have taken place
- Copies of the relevant medical/nursing records
- Any additional documentation, for example, post-mortem reports, death certificates
- The names and position of the other assessor(s) and the panel members
- A contact name and telephone number of the person at the Trust who is co-ordinating the review.

The preliminary report

After receiving the papers each clinical assessor should review the papers and evaluate whether:

- Any additional papers will be required
- It will be necessary to physically examine the patient prior to the Independent Review Panel
- Any equipment will be required on the day of the panel, for example X-ray viewing boxes
- They will need to see any part of the hospital prior to the panel, for example, the ward lay out
- Who they would like to interview at the Independent Review Panel.

Increasingly, panels are asking clinical assessors to produce a preliminary report, which is made available only to the panel, prior to the Independent Review Panel. This report should be based on the written information only. The reasons for the preliminary reports are to:

- Aid the panel and help them to understand the clinical aspects of the case
- Indicate whether there are any differences of clinical practice between the assessors

- Enable the panel members to identify areas of the complaint that may require clarification.

The suggested content of the preliminary report would be a summary of the clinical aspects of the case, bearing in mind the terms of reference. The findings and any recommendations should be listed under each of the terms of reference. Recommendations should be based on ways that will improve the effectiveness and efficiency of the service provided for future patients. It is important that the recommendations do not suggest disciplinary action as it is clearly indicated in the underpinning legislation that the panel cannot make recommendations about disciplinary action. The report will be read by lay people and should therefore concentrate on the clinical aspects of the terms of reference. Wherever possible, abbreviations should be avoided and any medical terms explained. It is also helpful to explain why a particular course of action or treatment was (or was not) taken.

The preliminary report should be sent to the Trust to be circulated to the panel members, this will enable the members to read the report and formulate any questions that they may wish to ask on its contents.

At the Independent Review Panel

It is becoming increasingly common for the panel members and clinical assessors to meet for about an hour immediately prior to the Independent Review Panel. This enables the members to meet each other and the panel members to question the clinical assessors on any areas of the complaint they do not understand and to clarify issues that may have arisen from the reports. In addition, the lay chair is able to indicate which areas of the complaint the panel members and the clinical assessors should lead on and establish the order of the questioning and the method of working of the panel.

During the Independent Review Panel hearing it is usual for the clinical assessors to take the lead on the clinical aspects of the complaint, both when the complainant and the complained against are being interviewed. Many lay chairs allow the complainant to ask the clinical assessors for explanations and clarification about certain aspects of the complaint; the panel members and the lay chair can also ask the clinical assessors to explain clinical issues. Care must be taken to ensure that both parties are treated equally and fairly.

A trend is now emerging that immediately after the Independent Review Panel, the panel members and the clinical assessors meet to decide the findings of fact and any recommendations that the panel may wish to make. This course of action makes the final report truly a panel report, and not just the view of one individual. If preliminary reports have been produced it is sometimes possible for the clinical assessors to then dictate

secondary care

2

their final report, which can either be a joint report or individual reports. The final report(s) will be appended to the panel's report and will therefore be seen by the patient. The report(s) should therefore be checked again to ensure that appropriate language is used and that they do not contain information that could cause 'serious harm' to the patient. It is helpful to the panel if the assessor's reports are produced as quickly as possible after the Independent Review Panel, as it is not possible to finalise the panel's report until the assessor's report(s) have been received.

STAFF SUPPORT

Staff are often adversely affected by being on the receiving end of a complaint. It is not unusual for them to report stress and sleepless nights. However, many try to cover up their stress, which may show in the form of aggression or simply ignoring the complaint and hoping it will go away. In extreme cases, staff may take time off sick when the effect of a complaint adds to the stress of a busy workload. Occupational Health, the Medical Defence Union and the Medical Protection Society all offer help and support. Information on how they can be contacted should be freely available to all staff. People do not forget if a complaint has been made against them and many can recall the incident in vivid detail many years after the original complaint has been dealt with.

Senior staff and managers should be aware of the effects that complaints have on staff and should be prepared to support them and to advise on external sources of support if appropriate.

Initially, complaints should always be discussed with individual staff members in private and care should be taken to listen to the member of staff's side of events before any judgements are made. The listening time given to staff at this stage can be invaluable in supporting them during this period. If junior staff have to attend meetings, a more senior member of staff should take time to explain the process fully and may, if appropriate, accompany them to give support.

21

The Health Service Commissioner in secondary care

Each year the Health Service Commissioner (the Ombudsman) produces an annual report, commenting on the previous year's work and outlining lessons that can be learned through the complaints system. He indicates areas of concern and potential areas where complaints can be prevented. In addition, he publishes information and reports on cases that have been investigated, usually at quarterly intervals. The reports are also available on the internet and are therefore easily accessible. This chapter considers the key messages coming out of the Ombudsman's reports with regard to secondary care and Health Authority complaints.

The theme running through the reports is that the Ombudsman has to decide if a member of staff's actions have been fair and reasonable, and that they are consistent with that of their peers.

ISSUES RAISED IN THE OMBUDSMAN'S REPORTS

Communication

To be efficient as a team it is important that the hospital staff communicate fully and effectively with each other and with the patient and their relatives. To enable this to happen, full and complete records should be kept. Records should be made of all communications relating to patient care and this should include a note of telephone conversations. The date and time that actions and communications have taken place, along with a clear indication about who is doing the recording, is important. Often, it is only by looking at patient's records that staff can demonstrate that they have acted competently and professionally.

Diagnostic testing

Unfortunately, some patients and relatives believe that a full range of diagnostic tests should be done. They believe that by not doing these tests the staff are failing to treat the patient appropriately. People who are requesting inappropriate, additional tests should be told why the tests are not applicable and, if they carry risks, what these are. Some complainants do not understand the terms 'false positive' and 'false negative' and, again, these require an explanation in lay terms.

Consent for treatment

The reports indicate problems and misunderstandings around the area of consent with regard to both the patients and their relatives.

There is confusion around the fact that patients have the right to refuse to undergo a particular treatment but that they do not have the right to demand a specific treatment. If the patient is unable to give consent, it is usual for the relatives to be consulted and to discuss the treatment that is offered. When consulting with relatives, doctors should not give the impression that they are obtaining permission for treatment from the relatives, as the relatives would neither have the right nor the responsibility to either give or withhold consent. Ultimately, the decision about the type of treatment given rests with the doctor and it is up to them to decide what action is to be taken.

Early discharge

If a patient is discharged from a hospital and then their condition alters so that they have to be readmitted there may be a complaint that the patient was discharged too soon. It is very easy to look at such cases and to decide that, with hindsight, the patient should not have been discharged. When examining such cases the Ombudsman would consider what was reasonable at the time of the discharge and would not take into consideration what subsequently happened.

Bereavement

A large number of complaints concern the care and treatment of patients who have subsequently died. Many relatives have the perception that an incorrect or late diagnosis may have contributed to the death. In other cases, there is concern over the decision not to resuscitate or not to continue active treatment. These complaints demonstrate the importance of clear communication with relatives, with clear explanation as to why a specific course of action is being taken or why it was not possible to make an earlier diagnosis.

Relatives as carers

The issues around the involvement of carers need careful and sensitive handling. Some relatives wish to be involved in the care of a loved one but others can feel pressurised and feel that they have to become involved, for example, if they think there is a shortage of nurses. Some relatives have unrealistic expectations about what is required of them and therefore good communication and clear and full record keeping is essential.

Nursing issues

Nursing complaints tend to be around the areas of the prevention and treatment of pressure sores, hygiene, the provision of food and fluid and delays in gaining the attention of ward staff.

All the above issues underline the importance of good communication and record keeping so that staff are able to clearly demonstrate what action has been taken, and when.

The Convening Decision

Unfortunately, some conveners fail to take clinical advice and do not consult with lay chairs at the Convening Decision stage. The regulations clearly state that, although the convener is responsible for the final decision, consultation must take place. It is also important that conveners and lay chairs do not investigate complaints.

Independent Review Panels

There is a degree of flexibility when conducting Independent Review Panels but it is still important to ensure that they fulfil the requirements of fairness and natural justice. Care must be taken to ensure that evidence is taken from key witnesses, from both parties to the complaint and, when clinical issues are discussed, that the clinical assessors are present.

secondary care

Appendix

Appendix: Department of Health Information and Guidance

LEGAL FRAMEWORK

Article 15(6), Directions to NHS Trusts, Health Authorities and Special Health Authorities for special hospitals on hospital complaints procedures.
Directions to Health Authorities on dealing with complaints about Family Health Services Practitioners.
Miscellaneous directions to Health Authorities for dealing with complaints.
The National Health Service (General Medical Services) amendment Regulations 1996 No. 702, Statutory Instrument.

GUIDANCE

Complaints – listening ... acting ... improving: Guidance on implementation of the NHS complaints procedure, issued 12 March 1996 under cover of EL(96)19.
Practice-based complaints procedures: Guidance for general practices, issued March 1996.
Travelling and other allowances for members of NHS Boards HSG(96)42.

HEALTH SERVICE CIRCULARS

Personal liability of non-executive directors of NHS Trusts, non-executive members of Health Authorities and non-executives of special Health Authorities. Serial number HSC 1998/010.
Personal liability of non-executives: Amendment of indemnity. Serial number HSC 1999/104.
Caldicott Guardians. Serial number HSC 1999/012.
For the record. Serial number HSC 1999/05.
Personal liability of non-executive directors of NHS Trusts, non-executive members of Health Authorities and non-executive directors of special Health Authorities. Serial number HSC 1998/010.
NHS complaints procedures: Confidentiality. Serial number HSC 1998/059.

EXECUTIVE LETTERS

Implementation of new complaints procedure: Final guidance EL(96) 19.
Payment of travelling and other allowances to chairmen, non-executive directors and members of committees and sub-committees of NHS Trusts. Issued by Head of Employment Issues NHS Executive, September 1996.

Family health services: Additional guidance on implementation of the NHS complaints procedure, FHSL(96)45: Annex.
Directions to Health Authorities on dealing with complaints about Family Health Service Practitioners, FHSL(97)24: Annex.

INTERNET INFORMATION

London Bereavement Network – www.bereavement.demon.co.uk/lbn/reading.html
Patient and Family Fact Sheets – www.cancer.org/rig/riggrief.html
Mental Health Net – Bereavement – www.mentalhelp.net/disorders/sx39.htm
Death of a child – www.compassionatefriends.com/respond.htm
The Health Service Commissioner – www.ombudsman.co.uk
Suggestions for Medical Personnel – www.compassionatefriends.com/medical.htm
The National Register of Public Service Interpreters – http://www.iol.org.uk

Mental Health Act

www.userguide.inuk.com

ADDRESSES

Association of Community Health Councils for England and Wales
(ACHCEW), Earlsmead House, 30 Drayton Park, London N5 1PB
Tel. 020 7609 8405
Institute of Linguists, Saxon House, 48 Southwark Street, London SE1 1UN
Tel. 020 7940 3100 Fax 0207 940 3101
Council on Tribunals, 22 Kingsway, London WC2B 6LE
Tel. 020 7936 7045
The Data Protection Registrar, Wycliffe House, Water Lane, Wilmslow, Cheshire SK9 5AF
Tel. 01625 545 745 (for information); tel. 01625 545 700 (switchboard)
Fax 01625 524 510
e-mail data@wycliffe.demon.co.uk
The Health Service Ombudsman, Millbank Tower, Millbank,
London SW1P 4QP
Tel. 020 7217 4051
The Medical Protection Society, 33 Cavendish Square, London W1N OPS
Tel. 020 7399 1300
The Medical Defence Union, 3 Devonshire Place, London W1N 2EA
Tel. 020 7486 6181
The General Dental Council, 37 Wimpole Street, London WlM 8OQ
Tel. 020 7887 3800

Further reading

EVALUATION OF THE COMPLAINTS SYSTEM

Which Magazine, September 1997, Cause for complaint
Which Magazine, September 1997, The complaints procedure
Wallace H, Mulcahy L 1999 Cause for complaint? The Public Law Project

COMMUNICATING BAD NEWS

Dear S 1995 Breaking bad news: caring for the family. Nursing Standard, December 6, 10(11)
Eden OB, Black I, MacKinlay GA, Emery AEH 1994 Communication with parents of children with cancer. Palliative Medicine 8: 105–114
Fallowfield L 1993 Giving sad and bad news. The Lancet 341: Feb 20
Morton R 1996 Breaking bad news to patients with cancer. Professional Nurse (11)10
Nottingham Local Medical Committee 1994 Difficult patients
O'Donovan S 1999 Reflections on breaking news of a family death. Nursing Times Nov 10, 95(44)
Parathian AR, Taylor F 1993 Can we insulate trainee nurses from exposure to bad practice? A study of role play in communicating bad news to patients. The Lancet 18: 801–807
Placek JT 1996 Breaking bad news, a review of the literature. JAMA August 14, 276(6)
Sanders CM 1992 Surviving Grief. John Wiley
Scorer CG 1980 Talking with patients. In: Vale A (ed) Medicine and the Christian mind, 2nd edn. Christian Medical Fellowship, London, pp 59–63
Sharp MC, Strauss RP, Lorch SC 1992 Communicating medical bad news: parent's experiences and preferences. The Journal of Pediatrics, 539–546
Sharp MC, Strauss RP, Lorch SC, Kachalia B 1995 Physicians and the communication of 'bad news': parent experiences of being informed of their child's cleft lip and/or palate. Pediatrics 96(1): 82–89
Wilner Gale 1997 Vexatious complainants, The Associate, National Association of Complaints Personnel, Health, Volume 1.2
Zunin LM, Zunin HS 1991 The art of condolence. Harper Perennial

THE HEALTH SERVICE COMMISSIONER'S OFFICE

Health Service Commissioner 1999 Annual Report 1998–1999
Health Service Commissioner 1999 Investigations completed October 1998 to March 1999
Health Service Commissioner 1999 Investigation of complaints about clinical failings
Health Service Commissioner 1999 Investigations about aspects of the NHS complaints procedure

Health Service Commissioner 1999 Investigation of complaints about treatment by deputising doctors and monitoring of a GP deputising service
Health Service Commissioner 1998 Investigations completed April to September 1998
Health Service Commissioner 1998 Annual Report 1997–1998
Health Service Commissioner 1998 Investigations completed October 1997 to March 1998

Personal communications

COMMUNICATING BAD NEWS

Bennett R, Hospital Chaplain, Bassetlaw NHS Trust

MENTAL HEALTH

Child A, Director of Nursing, Northumberland Mental Health NHS Trust
Read E, Consumer Relations Manager, Nottingham Healthcare NHS Trust

INTERPRETERS

Corsellis A, Professional interpreter, Institute of Linguists

COMMUNITY HEALTH COUNCILS

Smith M, Chief Officer, Bassetlaw Community Health Council

THE HEALTH SERVICE COMMISSIONER'S OFFICE

Drake E, Investigations Manager, Health Service Commissioner's office

Index

Index